THE UNIQUE PARENT
Club

Navigating the Extraordinary Journey
of Special Needs Parenting

KATHLEEN BROWNE

First published by Ultimate World Publishing 2024
Copyright © 2024 @kathleenbrowne

ISBN

Paperback: 978-1-923123-98-4
Ebook: 978-1-923123-99-1

@kathleenbrowne has asserted her rights under the Copyright, Designs and Patents Act 1988 to be identified as the author of this work. The information in this book is based on the author's experiences and opinions. The publisher specifically disclaims responsibility for any adverse consequences which may result from use of the information contained herein. Permission to use information has been sought by the author. Any breaches will be rectified in further editions of the book.

All rights reserved. No part of this publication may be reproduced, stored in or introduced into a retrieval system, or transmitted in any form, or by any means (electronic, mechanical, photocopying, recording or otherwise) without the prior written permission of the author. Any person who does any unauthorised act in relation to this publication may be liable to criminal prosecution and civil claims for damages. Enquiries should be made through the publisher.

Cover design: Ultimate World Publishing
Layout and typesetting: Ultimate World Publishing
Editor: Vanessa McKay
Photo credit: Keegan Browne and Joan Tatchell

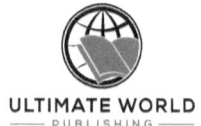

Ultimate World Publishing
Diamond Creek,
Victoria Australia 3089
www.writeabook.com.au

Dedication

This book is dedicated to everyone in my family. Family, the cornerstone of my existence, has been the wellspring of inspiration and support throughout my life. Each member has left an indelible mark, shaping the person I am today. In this chapter, I want to pay homage to those who have played pivotal roles in my journey, starting with my late mother.

My late mother, Bridget Dorothy Morrow-Tatchell, was my shining light, my unique guide, who gave me strength when I felt I couldn't go on. Her wisdom and love were my constant companions, and her memory continues to be a source of inspiration for me. She taught me to persevere, to find strength in adversity, and to love unconditionally. This book is a tribute to her enduring legacy, a testament to the profound impact she had on my life.

I dedicate this part to the memory of my late husband, Gerald Ivor Browne, a pillar of unwavering support during our shared journey through life. He was the one who always said, "he will be fine," even when things were tough. His words of encouragement served as a beacon of hope during the darkest hours, and his memory remains a source of strength. This book is a tribute to his unshakeable faith and his enduring love, which continues to guide me even in his absence.

You, my son Keegan Matthew, have opened my eyes to so many things that I may not have known otherwise. Your presence in my life has been a source of boundless joy and a reminder of the beauty that the world offers. With each passing day, you inspire me to embrace life's wonders and to cherish the moments we share. This book is a testament to the love and gratitude I feel for you.

I will always be grateful to my son Bradlee Dean for his selflessness and his unwavering support. He has undertaken countless acts of kindness, not only for me but also for his brother Keegan. His love for you, Keegan, knows no bounds, and his dedication to our family has been unwavering. This book is a tribute to the strength and unity that binds us as a family, thanks to Bradlee's unending love and support.

To my siblings and in-laws, I extend my heartfelt thanks for your support over the years. Your presence in my life has enriched it in countless ways, and I am deeply grateful for the bonds we share. This book is a recognition of the collective love and support that has sustained me throughout my journey.

I extend heartfelt dedication and gratitude to the countless medical professionals from South Africa, New Zealand, and Australia who have played an extraordinary role in Keegan's and my life. Although I may not recall your names individually, your impact on our lives is immeasurable.

Dedication

Thank you for your unwavering dedication and the countless times you stepped in to provide crucial medical interventions that have kept Keegan healthy. The nurses, doctors, and allied health professionals have gone above and beyond, offering specialised services that have been instrumental in Keegan's well-being. Your commitment to your profession has made a profound difference; I am eternally grateful.

I am dedicating this book to my family, who have been the foundation upon which my life's story has been built, and their influence will continue to shape the chapters ahead. My book celebrates love, resilience, and enduring ties that make us who we are.

Contents

Dedication	iii
Introduction	1
Chapter 1: Entry To The Unique Parent Club	3
Chapter 2: Grasping The Emotional Storm After Your Child's Diagnosis	13
Chapter 3: Diagnosis	25
Chapter 4: Engaging Therapies Early	39
Chapter 5: Advocacy	45
Chapter 6: Education	51
Chapter 7: Building a Support Network	59
Chapter 8: Managing The Emotional Rollercoaster	69
Chapter 9: Resilient Mum, Single Carer, Social Worker, And Ndis Registered Provider	75
Chapter 10: Balancing Work And Parenting	85
Chapter 11: Celebrating Milestones And Success	93
Chapter 12: Future Planning	101
Chapter 13: Life Lessons Learned	113
About The Author	125
Join The Unique Parent Club With Kathleen Browne	127
The Unique Parent Club	131
A Parenting Coaching Program	135
Resources	139

Introduction

Welcome to The Unique Parent Club, a heartfelt guide crafted for those who have embarked upon the extraordinary journey of special needs parenting. Authored by Kathleen Browne, this book is a compassionate companion, offering wisdom, insights, and unwavering support to those navigating the unique challenges and joys of raising exceptional children.

In The Unique Parent Club, Kathleen draws upon her experiences, transforming them into a beacon of hope for parents in uncharted territory. With a blend of warmth and candour, she shares the highs and lows of her journey, creating a tapestry of understanding that resonates with the diverse spectrum of special needs parenting.

As a member of The Unique Parent Club, you are not alone. Kathleen invites you into a community bound by shared experiences and everyday triumphs. Through this book, she extends a helping hand, offering practical advice, emotional solace, and a roadmap for navigating the intricacies of advocating for and nurturing children with special needs.

The Unique Parent Club is not just a guide; it's an invitation to embrace the extraordinary. Kathleen's words empower parents to celebrate the uniqueness of their children, fostering an environment where differences are not just accepted but cherished. This book is a testament to the strength, resilience, and boundless love that defines the members of The Unique Parent Club.

Embark on this transformative journey with Kathleen Browne as your guide, and discover the extraordinary beauty of being a part of The Unique Parent Club. Together, let us navigate the challenges, celebrate the victories, and embrace the richness that special needs parenting brings to our lives.

CHAPTER 1

Entry To The Unique Parent Club

I always believed that joining a club was a choice, but as a new parent to a child with special needs, it felt like I had no choice. Surprisingly, this lack of choice made me part of an inclusive community. I wish all parents of children with special needs would realise the uniqueness of their situation and find joy in parenting their extraordinary child.

On a chilly Wednesday morning, the first day of February 1989, I found myself wrestling with excruciating stomach pains. Carrying my first child, I wasn't taking any chances. With my late husband by my side, we casually strolled to my gynecologist's office. A thorough examination led to a clear directive – head straight to the hospital. Our baby was poised to make an entrance into the world on this very day. Today! My response of disbelief lingered in the air, countered by the doctor's assertive statement: "Yes, today." And so, armed with uncertainty about the labour journey, we embarked on the road to Mary Mount Hospital. The pain intensified with each passing moment.

I was eight months pregnant, utterly bewildered. This revelation hit me like a lightning bolt on the first day of my eagerly awaited maternity leave. The due date I had carefully marked on my calendar, March 1st, 1989, had somehow morphed into February 1st, 1989. A wave of disbelief swept through me – had I miscalculated the conception date of my baby?

Panic set in as I grappled with the notion of an unexpectedly early arrival. My detailed plans were tailored for a March delivery, and the possibility of a February birth caught me completely off guard. Enduring the agonising waves of pain, punctuated by the doctor's directives and my own screams, I was thrust into a whirlwind of chaos.

In the midst of labour, my late husband, a constant presence throughout my pregnancy, posed the question again – his recurring inquiry about waiting outside the delivery room. My response remained unwavering, a resolute, "yes." His figure in green swiftly disappeared from my view as he exited the delivery suite, leaving me alone with my thoughts and the imminent arrival.

Only a nurse accompanied me as the obstetrician appeared in the delivery suite. My late husband, obscured by the green gown, had vanished, his giant strides echoing in my ears. It was a deliberate choice for him to stay out; in the throes of pain, I preferred solitude. Unwanted attention only heightened my discomfort, and in those moments, no one but me or medication held the power to alleviate the pain.

With the arrival of our baby, the room echoed with a chorus of cries. The tiny bundle had a fleeting moment on my chest before being swiftly taken to the hospital nursery. The nurse and doctor carried out their tasks, ensuring my well-being before giving the green light for our transfer to the hospital maternity ward. And so, amid the whirlwind of emotions and pain, the journey into motherhood commenced, marked by unforeseen turns and a silent understanding between my late husband and me.

The Initiation into the Unique Parent Club unfolded. Twenty-four hours post-birth, I had just finished breastfeeding when my son was returned to the nursery to join other newborns. In 1989, it was customary for mothers to have time for rest and recovery after childbirth. The hospital nurseries played a crucial role during this period, caring for our babies until we were ready to feed, bathe, and spend wakeful moments with them. Our little ones peacefully slept in the nursery for the remaining time, offering us the precious moments needed for recuperation.

On a Thursday morning, the second day of February 1989, I lay in my hospital bed when a doctor approached. Introducing himself as the hospital pediatrician, he explained he had examined my baby, revealing something unusual – webbed fingers, toes, and a single line across his palm. I felt my body tremble, instinctively seeking refuge under the blanket as if it could shield me from the unexpected.

Curiosity led me to ask how the doctor had noticed these features. He recounted being called to examine my baby because of the absence of bowel movements within the first twenty-four hours. Though Down syndrome wasn't confirmed, concerns arose about a possible blockage. The doctor explained that six weeks were needed to confirm a Down syndrome diagnosis, with additional medical procedures required to determine the cause of the bowel issue.

And thus began my extraordinary journey, steering me down the winding path of special needs parenting, navigating highs and lows with courage and determination.

Feeling powerless, my late husband arrived at Mary Mount Hospital. Within minutes, documents to transfer our newborn to Brenthurst Clinic were signed. Together in an ambulance, we transitioned to a new hospital. Although urged to stay in the ward until formally discharged, I declined, opting not to be separated from my baby.

Tears, worry, and questions persisted. I cried so much that my tears seemed to dry up at some point. My late husband's shock manifested differently; he remained silent, staring into space, grappling with questions like how and what do we do. The absence of answers left us consoling each other based on the doctor's diagnosis of our son's medical condition.

<u>Stress has a way of dulling your senses</u>. My late husband and I were in a whirlwind of consultations with doctors, surgeons, specialists, nurses, nuns, and fellow parents in the children's hospital ward. There was no shortage of company; just when you thought you could take a moment to breathe, someone else arrived to chat, especially when I was alone at the hospital.

The doctors summoned my late husband and me on the second day at the new hospital, Brenthurst Clinic. They delivered the news that our son had a blockage in his bowel. Their plan was to continue efforts to help him pass stool through his bowel; if unsuccessful, surgery would be necessary. The doctor mentioned the likelihood of a medical condition called Hirschsprung's Disease. I asked, "What is that?" The term was entirely unfamiliar, and the doctor explained that some of my son's bowels lacked muscle tone, a common trait in boys and those with Down syndrome. Now, in addition to Down syndrome, we were grappling with Hirschsprung's Disease, low muscle tone, bowel obstruction, an irregular heartbeat, known as a heart murmur, and who knew what else. The doctor tried to guide us through this new information, even writing the name of the disease on paper so we wouldn't forget. It felt like there was no turning back.

The doctors weren't done; they continued unveiling issues with my baby. According to them, he didn't have a normal palate. A deep ridge in his palate hindered proper sucking, prompting an instant placement of a tube in his nose to ensure he received the necessary nutrients. And it didn't end there.

The doctors also mentioned that my baby's tongue was enlarged. What did that mean? Apparently, it was common for babies with Down syndrome to have an enlarged tongue, and they cautioned that he might not be able to close his mouth. Just when I thought it couldn't get more overwhelming, it did. At some point, I thought it might help to pray for my baby. Prayer was my last resort, a familiar solace from my Catholic upbringing. Silently, I prayed not just for my child but for all the children in the hospital ward, for my late husband and me, hoping we could find the strength to endure what lay ahead.

<u>Prayer became my refuge</u> as I fervently wished for my baby's survival and well-being, irrespective of his condition. At that moment, all I craved was for him to live so I could fulfil my role as a mother and care for him. The doctors couldn't provide more information, and my overwhelmed mind forced me to take a break, grappling with self-blame for my baby's condition.

On the third day of my son's life, I was engrossed in reading by his incubator. A nun, dressed in traditional attire and carrying books and her bag, approached me. She identified herself and explained her visit was to pray for my baby, given his Catholic designation on the hospital admission. Grateful for any prayers, I welcomed her kind offer.

After her prayer, she suggested baptising my baby while in the hospital. My immediate response was to ask if she thought my child was going to die. Her answer was no, but she pointed out his severe illness. Unsettled by her suggestion, I firmly stated that my child would be baptised when he was well and when I felt ready. The nun, taken aback, apologised, acknowledging that I could choose the timing of the baptism.

Amidst my despair and uncertainty, prayer became a lifeline. It was a desperate plea, an emotional overflow of my deepest fears and hopes. As a new mother, my sole desire was for my baby to not only survive but thrive, regardless of the challenges ahead. I longed to be there for him, navigating the joys and struggles of motherhood.

Standing in that sterile hospital room, I sought answers from the doctors, yearning for words that would ease the overwhelming burden on my shoulders. However, information was elusive, and my mind, burdened by the gravity of the situation, shut down. It felt like being thrust into a nightmarish world of uncertainty, and guilt became the prevailing emotion.

In those early days of motherhood, I discovered that prayer alone couldn't erase the challenges ahead. Nevertheless, it served as a lifeline, a means to articulate my hopes and fears and a wellspring of strength in the face of uncertainty. The journey was far from over, but armed with unwavering determination and a mother's boundless love, I was ready to embrace whatever lay ahead.

The fourth day weighed heavily on me. As I entered the hospital, it marked the fourth day of our harrowing journey with our baby. Stepping into the children's ward, my eyes anxiously searched the room, but my baby was nowhere to be seen. Frozen in place, I couldn't muster the strength to move. My heart raced as I noticed a nurse at her workstation. Sensing my distress, she quickly rose from her chair and hastened towards me. She explained she had been trying to reach me by phone but couldn't – it was 1989, and our apartment lacked a landline phone, and mobile phones were still nonexistent.

She guided me to the waiting room with a swift and reassuring gesture. There, a pediatric nurse met me and delivered the news that sent shivers down my spine: my baby's bowel had burst, necessitating immediate surgery. The plan was to remove the part of his bowel lacking muscle and reattach the healthy portions, ensuring he could pass stool.

My baby was undergoing surgery at that very moment, a process that would demand four agonising hours of waiting patiently to hear the doctor confirm his survival. Having not witnessed him being wheeled into the theatre, my imagination painted a picture of this tiny, four-day-old baby in his incubator, navigating the hospital corridors on his way to the operating theatre, his fate uncertain.

Guilt once again consumed me as I grappled with not being at his bedside day and night. Yet, my thoughts returned to the nurse's and doctor's assurances, urging me to care for myself and assuring me that my baby was in capable hands. Despite following their guidance, the guilt of not being present when my baby needed me most lingered.

My focus shifted to notifying family members about my baby's surgery. My late husband had gone to work that day, deeming it unnecessary for us to continuously sit and watch over our baby. Upon hearing the news of our baby's surgery, he rushed to the hospital to provide support. The waiting room transformed into a space of profound tension and anxiety. Silence enveloped the room, broken only by my repeated mantra, "We will get through this; my baby will get through this." It wouldn't be easy for him, but I believed he would make it.

And so, my little warrior emerged victorious from his life-saving surgery. There he lay, nestled in an incubator, half his tiny head shorn of hair, an intricate web of tubes emerging from him. A feeding tube delicately snaked into his nose, and the doctor explained the need for a small incision in his little arm for a drip, a challenge in finding a vein. Yet, amidst the array of tubes—breathing, feeding, and the drip—it was a relief to know that my baby had triumphed over the surgery, bravely embracing the tools of recovery.

Initially, I failed to notice changes in his little belly, still adorned with a diaper. The bag on his stomach escaped my attention as my focus centred on his face and expressions, trying to gauge his comfort amidst the tubes. Then, the doctor called us to the waiting room, delivering the startling news – our baby required major surgery. About four centimetres of his bowel lacked muscle, and the doctor needed to remove and stitch everything back together for him to have a regular bowel movement. The gravity of the situation hit us hard.

Our baby's surgeon, a compassionate and seasoned Medical Professor, donned a charming little bow tie. His wealth of experience exuded confidence as he explained the necessity of creating a stoma surgically. Placed on the baby's stomach, the stoma allowed him to pass stool into a colostomy bag. The concept of a colostomy bag was entirely new. It struck fear into our hearts, raising concerns about its impact on our child's current and future well-being.

In a candid conversation, the doctor assured us that the colostomy bag was a temporary solution. Our baby wouldn't have to rely on it for life, but the uncertainty lay in not knowing when it could be removed. It became a waiting game, demanding patience to navigate these challenging moments.

Amidst these challenges, we sat by the incubator, unable to hold our baby for the initial eight days of his life. Each morning, we awaited updates from the nurses on his medical progress, engaging in consultations with doctors, the Medical Professor, nurses, and allied health professionals. Support from family and friends proved invaluable during this tumultuous journey.

One vivid memory is the Medical Professor's unique morning ritual, as he warmly greeted parents before checking on his special tiny patient. His greetings, infused with humour, created a distinctive connection with our baby. He'd say, "Hello, sausage, how's your colostomy?" While my late husband may not have entirely embraced the doctor's unorthodox greeting, for me, it provided a welcomed break from the stress and constant care demanded by our baby's condition. The nickname 'sausage' stuck around, adding a touch of lightness to this challenging chapter in our lives.

Endearingly nicknamed Dr. Bowtie, he became a constant presence in our lives, gracing us with daily visits until our baby's discharge. Dr. Bowtie holds a special place in our hearts because, amidst the challenges, he was uniquely able to bring a smile to my face during those trying days.

The key takeaway from our experience <u>was embracing the entry into The Unique Parents Club.</u> This initiation marked a significant moment, propelling us into a community that brought both challenges and excitement. As we welcomed our ten-day-old baby home, a mix of emotions—nervousness, happiness, fear, and excitement—defined our journey as new parents.

Despite the uncertainty of parenthood, we recognised that this unique journey was both daunting and full of promise, shaping our path in the ever-evolving adventure of being parents.

CHAPTER 2

Grasping The Emotional Storm After Your Child's Diagnosis

The profound significance of naming a baby and adhering to our beliefs unfolded before me in ways I hadn't anticipated. As we embarked on the journey of baptising our son and selecting godparents, I was navigating through a tumultuous emotional storm that seemed to encompass the unpredictable elements of hail, rain, sun, and cloudbursts simultaneously. The juxtaposition of these sacred rituals with the internal tempest underscored the depth of the emotional journey that parenthood can unexpectedly bring.

BABY NAMING

Registering our baby's birth turned out to be quite a puzzle. Picture this: you've anticipated a baby girl for months, only to find yourself contemplating what to name a baby boy. My late husband was convinced we were having a daughter, and I deliberately chose not to discover the baby's sex beforehand. For me, the gender didn't matter as long as the baby was healthy. We did not expect our surprise to arrive as a 3.75-kilogram baby boy with the most adorable rosy chubby cheeks.

Choosing a name became a task of careful consideration. My late husband and I exchanged ideas on the perfect name for our newborn son. After much contemplation, we settled on the name Keegan Matthew Browne. The name seemed to fit him seamlessly from the day we gave it to him, and it continues to suit him perfectly.

Yet Keegan's name has undergone a transformation over time. Although officially known as Keegan, our family has coined various endearing nicknames for him. 'Sausage', 'Keeg', 'Humphrey', 'Humfs', and 'Chap', are just a few of the affectionate terms we've playfully attached to him. Surprisingly, Keegan embraces these nicknames, and more often than not, he responds to the name 'Humphrey.' He's aware of his given name and keenly understands when to acknowledge it. When I address him as 'Keegan Matthew Browne,' he typically ignores me, a quirk I've learned to accept, hoping for the best.

CONFIRMATION OF DIAGNOSIS

Our journey with Keegan took an unexpected turn when, at six weeks old, he received a diagnosis of Down Syndrome and Hirschsprung's Disease. At that point, he had already been discharged from the hospital and was back home with us. While the diagnosis wasn't entirely surprising, it marked the commencement of a new chapter in our lives. We understood that more surgeries and challenges lay ahead but were resolute in confronting them head-on. Keegan's strength and resilience served as a testament to the extraordinary spirit within him, destined to inspire us all even on the day of his baptism.

BAPTISING KEEGAN

Baptising Keegan was a poignant moment in our parenthood journey. With carefully chosen godparents and a baby showing signs of resilience, the sacred ceremony unfolded. To our amusement, Keegan slept soundly, seemingly unaware of the profound significance. His newly shaved head stood as a symbolic testament to his strength and the enveloping love surrounding him.

While Keegan was thriving in his own way, little did he know that his parents were navigating a unique journey. Venturing into parenthood for the first time while caring for a child with special needs felt like being on a rollercoaster with an uncertain end. We were yearning for it to stop, although we weren't quite sure why. The ambiguity surrounding what would happen when the ride halted added to the emotional complexity.

During this tumultuous time, unanswered questions multiplied. Uncertainty left me grappling with a mix of emotions, unsure of how to feel, think, or act on certain days. Amidst the turmoil, the only constant was the reminder to maintain faith—that both my baby and I would endure. Lacking a roadmap for this unfamiliar terrain, I pondered whether others had trod this path before. What did those parents do? How did they navigate the challenges, and where did they find the answers we desperately sought?

FACING UNEXPECTED CHALLENGES

Feeling utterly unprepared, I grappled with the absence of a roadmap for this uncharted territory. From changing Keegan's colostomy bag to ensuring he consumed the right amount of food, every task felt like uncharted territory. The unexpected challenge of dealing with the gas from the colostomy bag left me utterly unprepared – a sentiment I can only describe as horrendous.

Changing Keegan in Public Places: A Humorous, Embarrassing, and Unforgettable Episode

Keegan, only a few weeks old, accompanied me to a routine doctor's appointment, setting the stage for a moment that was equal parts funny, embarrassing, and downright challenging for those in close proximity. Keegan's colostomy bag, a constant companion since he was four days old, played a pivotal role in this memorable event. This specialised bag collected his stool when he passed gas, and it encircled the stoma on his stomach.

On this day, Keegan was unusually windy. The colostomy bag visibly inflated each time he released gas, creating a real-time demonstration of his digestive activity. As his bag expanded, my duty as a parent involved preventing it from bursting or dislodging by promptly releasing the accumulating air. So, in the midst of a doctor's appointment, I found myself managing Keegan's distinctive way of signalling that he was done with his business.

As I opened the bottom of the colostomy bag to release the air, an unmistakable odour began to permeate the entire doctor's room. The waiting patients exchanged puzzled glances, attempting to identify the source of the unexpected fragrance. At that moment, embarrassment overwhelmed me, and I struggled to apologise for my son's rather unconventional bowel movements. Opting for a composed facade, I mirrored the nonchalant expressions of the other parents in the room.

The distinct aroma, though unpleasant, seemed to defy the innocence of Keegan's small frame. Dr Bowtie humorously suggested the remedy of lighting a match to absorb the smell – a tactic perhaps suitable for home but not reasonably practical in doctor's offices, hospitals, baby clinics, public transport, or during visits to friends and family. The unexpected olfactory adventure became a memorable chapter in our parenting journey, a reminder that even the most routine tasks took on a uniquely adventurous twist with Keegan.

EMOTIONAL ROLLERCOASTER OF PARENTHOOD

While the journey with Keegan resembled a rollercoaster for everyone involved, as his mother, the twists and turns took on a unique meaning. My emotional spectrum expanded, and each bend brought forth a raft of sentiments, from grief to guilt, worry, financial concerns, and contemplation of long-term implications. Navigating the complex terrain of emotions became integral to my role as a mother, intertwining with the challenges and joys that characterised our parenting journey with Keegan.

NAVIGATING THE DEPTHS OF GRIEF

Grief was an unwelcome companion on this unexpected journey. It became a weight I grappled with as a mother. Each day brought forth its own set of challenges and waves of sorrow and longing with them. The grieving process extended beyond the perceived norms of parenthood, enveloping me in a complex dance of emotions. It was a profound struggle to reconcile the dreams I had envisioned for Keegan with the reality we faced. You feel sadness, loss, and hopelessness creeping into your head. I wasn't sure what to feel. Despite being happy, I was sad. In this grief, I found strength in embracing our path's uniqueness and cherishing the moments of resilience and joy that shone through the shadows of loss.

THE GUILT DILEMMA

I found myself ensnared in the trap of guilt, wrestling with self-blame for smoking and drinking during the early stages of my pregnancy, especially when I was unaware of my pregnancy. However, upon discovering that I was expecting, I took immediate action to cease smoking and abstain from alcohol to safeguard both my health and the well-being of my unborn baby. While grappling with hindsight regret, I also acknowledged the steps I had taken to prioritise the health of my child once I became aware of the pregnancy. The internal struggle between past actions and subsequent efforts to make amends became a complex facet of my journey into motherhood.

THE WEIGHT OF WORRY

The unrelenting grip of worry became a constant companion. This force could drain one's energy and divert attention from the present moment. My concerns for Keegan's health manifested as a cascade of questions that occupied my thoughts. Would he recover? Could he eventually walk, talk, make friends, and navigate the world's complexities? The uncertainty surrounding his future added an extra layer of weight to the already challenging journey, fostering a persistent sense of unease and prompting a continuous quest for reassurance.

NAVIGATING THE FINANCIAL CHALLENGES OF SPECIAL NEEDS PARENTING

One profound challenge in parenting a child with special needs is the unexpected financial expenses. The array of expenses, from medical bills to therapy costs and specialised equipment, swiftly accumulates, creating a strain on financial resources. The continuous juggling act involves ensuring that your child receives the necessary and the best care and maintaining a delicate balance within the confines of your budget. The financial aspect of this journey adds an extra layer of complexity, underscoring the need for resilience and strategic planning to meet the unique demands that come with caring for a child with special needs.

EMBARKING ON THE QUEST FOR MEDICAL FUNDS

Traversing the intricacies of the healthcare system and identifying the right medical funds to cater to the needs of a special needs child is a formidable undertaking. It can often feel like navigating an uphill terrain with challenges and complexities. Despite the arduous nature of the journey, it's a climb we willingly undertake, fueled by an unwavering commitment to securing the necessary resources for the optimal well-being of our children. In the face of this daunting task, the resilience and determination to navigate the intricacies of medical funding become paramount elements of the broader journey of caring for a child with special needs.

NAVIGATING THE UNCHARTED TERRITORY OF SPECIAL NEEDS PARENTHOOD

In the realm of parenting, where blueprints don't exist, my role extended beyond conventional parenthood—I was a special needs parent to a child with unique requirements. While acknowledging that all infants demand special attention and care, my focus inevitably honed in on my child's diagnosis and health.

Special needs parenting often involves forging uncharted paths and devising solutions tailored to the distinctive challenges that arise. There's no universal guide, and we find ourselves piecing together strategies as we navigate the unknown. In the absence of a blueprint, I grappled with feelings of fault as questions about the purpose behind my child's presence in my life and uncertainties about his future lingered.

Repeatedly, I asked:

Why were you given to me?

What lessons do I need to learn from you?

Who do you resemble?

What does the future hold for you?

Without clear answers, I forged ahead, recognising that the journey of special needs parenting is one where resilience, adaptability, and a willingness to embrace the unknown become indispensable companions.

THE WEIGHT OF SELF-BLAME AND QUESTIONS OF A HIGHER POWER

Every day, the burden of blame weighed heavily on my shoulders as I grappled with my son's birth defects. It seemed unfathomable to point fingers elsewhere when, in my mind, the responsibility squarely rested on me. The surgeries, the challenges with his colostomy bag, and the absence of a fully functional bowel all became facets of his struggle that I internalised as my own failings. The strength to shift blame onto someone else eluded me.

In moments of deep contemplation, I questioned whether I could lay blame on a higher power, on God. Was there a conceivable way to attribute responsibility to the divine, and if so, how could I navigate this path? The notion lingered in my thoughts as I grappled with the idea that perhaps God intended for me to endure suffering, learn profound lessons, and remain occupied by granting me a child with disabilities and numerous medical challenges. The constant pondering reflected the internal struggle to reconcile the concept of divine intent with my challenges in caring for my child and the introspective journey it catalysed.

THE WEIGHT OF GUILT AND THE UNANSWERED QUESTIONS

The guilt of blaming God left me frustrated, especially when my prayers seemed to echo in the silence with no response. Despite the frustration, assigning blame, even to a higher authority, felt like a way to redirect anger away from myself. I could release my frustrations into the ethereal realm, allowing my thoughts and prayers to float in the air, unheard by the divine.

However, vocalising my prayers, even aloud, brought no tangible change. The internal conflict persisted, and the unanswered questions lingered. Visitors, eager to find resemblance in the new baby, often inquired, "Who does he look like?" The consensus was that he resembled me due to a slightly lighter complexion than his dad. Yet, as his mother, I struggled to discern my features in him. He was a unique and handsome little individual, a pudding of his own. I couldn't pinpoint any specific familial resemblance, adding another layer to the complexity of my emotions and perceptions during that challenging time.

DISHEARTENING DOCTORS ADVICE

In the midst of navigating these challenging moments, I scheduled a six-week post-birth checkup with my gynecologist. This routine appointment, reminiscent of my experience with Keegan, involved a patient waiting for my turn, hoping for a clean bill of health after the birth of my baby. During the examination, my gynecologist reassured me that my body had healed without complications, a relief I welcomed wholeheartedly.

To my surprise, the doctor proceeded to share that he had examined Keegan on the day of his birth and detected nothing unusual about him—no signs of a potential disability. He emphasised that if there had been any concerns, he would have communicated them immediately. Then, he delved into a discussion about my age, deeming my youthfulness at twenty-six as an opportunity to consider placing my child in a specialised facility for children with disabilities. According to him, this would free me to pursue a more fulfilling life unburdened by the responsibilities of raising a child with special needs. This proposition left me utterly flabbergasted.

At that moment, I couldn't help but reflect on the fact that the doctor had initially missed diagnosing my child at birth. Who was he to suggest such a life-altering decision without genuinely understanding my capabilities and personal circumstances? Despite my bewilderment, I expressed gratitude for his input and chose not to return. It left me pondering how frequently he might have given similar advice to other parents facing the challenges of raising children with special needs.

I recognised that it was my responsibility to embrace the role of parenting Keegan fully. This meant immersing myself in understanding everything about him—his diagnosis, his health, and his overall well-being. My commitment was to ensure that he received the best care possible from both a young mother and father who cherished him deeply, allowing us all to find fulfilment in this unique journey.

CHAPTER 3

Diagnosis

Little did I know that I would embark on a journey to comprehend a multitude of medical terms, my child's diagnosis, and the intricacies of children's growth and development all at once. Gathering information on Down Syndrome Hirschsprung's Disease, caring for a stoma, and changing a colostomy bag became imperative. My crucial first step involved delving into the understanding of the diagnosis itself and what I needed to do to intervene and support my baby.

KEEGAN'S DIAGNOSIS AND THE SEARCH FOR UNDERSTANDING

The moment the doctors revealed that my son had Down Syndrome, an overwhelming surge of shock and guilt enveloped me. The weight of those words hit me like a ton of bricks, and my initial response was disbelief. How could this be happening? The journey of comprehension was fraught with emotions. Still, as time unfolded, the shock and guilt gradually subsided, and I began to come to terms with the reality.

Understanding Down Syndrome required a shift in my perspective. It wasn't a disease that had developed in my baby; instead, it was a genetic condition he had carried from the very beginning. This insight marked a turning point in my journey of acceptance. However, the road ahead was still obscured by questions about the consequences of this diagnosis.

For those unfamiliar with the specifics, Keegan has Down Syndrome, which is also referred to as Trisomy 21. Keegan was born with an additional copy of chromosome 21. Because of the extra chromosome, his genetic material led to his developmental delays, intellectual disability, and distinctive physical features. Down Syndrome, as I understood it, can occur in individuals of any race or socioeconomic background, which emphasises the random nature of this genetic condition.

THE COMPLEXITY OF TRISOMY 21

My son, Keegan, has Trisomy 21, a specific form of Down Syndrome, which meant he had an extra copy of chromosome 21. Understanding the implications of this genetic variation was a significant challenge for me. It necessitated a deep dive into learning about the condition, its potential effects, and how it would shape Keegan's life.

Trisomy 21 is characterised by certain physical features, such as almond-shaped eyes, a single crease across the palm of the hand, and a protruding tongue. While it can lead to various health issues, it's crucial to remember that every child's experience is unique.

THE CAUSE OF DOWN SYNDROME

One common question I often ask is what causes Trisomy 21. Medical science suggests that it typically results from a random error during the formation of sperm or egg cells, leading to an extra copy of chromosome 21. The exact cause remains unknown, but advancements in medical science have helped identify some risk factors.

In addition to Down Syndrome, Keegan was also diagnosed with Hirschsprung's Disease, a condition characterised by a deficiency of muscle tone in the colon, hindering the smooth passage of stool. To address this condition, a surgical procedure is typically performed, involving the creation of a stoma on the exterior part of the stomach to facilitate healing and bowel function. In Keegan's case, he underwent a significant surgical intervention where a portion of his bowel was removed, allowing the medical team to address and rectify his condition, ultimately enabling him to experience regular bowel movements and regain a sense of normalcy at a young age of nine months in his daily life. This procedure was vital in his journey toward improved health and well-being.

EARLY DIAGNOSIS AND MOVING FORWARD

Initially, when the doctors told me about Keegan's Down syndrome, they hadn't identified the specific Trisomy 21 variant. Their diagnosis primarily relied on physical features. However, further tests and examinations confirmed his unique genetic makeup.

Moving forward, my late husband and I had to transition from the initial shock to a learning phase. We needed to understand the specific challenges our child would face and how we, as a family, would navigate them.

UNDERSTANDING HIRSCHBRUNGS DISEASE

Hirschsprung's disease, also known as congenital aganglionic megacolon, is a rare genetic disorder that affects the large intestine (colon) and, in some cases, the rectum. The condition is characterised by the absence of nerve cells, called ganglion cells, in the lower part of the colon. These ganglion cells regulate the muscle contractions necessary for moving stool through the digestive tract. In individuals with Hirschsprung's disease, this absence of ganglion cells in a specific segment of the colon results in a blockage, preventing the normal passage of stool.

Hirschsprung's disease typically presents in newborns or infants and can lead to various symptoms, including Chronic Constipation. Babies with Hirschsprung's disease may experience severe constipation shortly after birth. They might have difficulty passing stool, leading to abdominal discomfort and bloating.

Abdominal Distension: The accumulation of stool in the blocked portion of the colon can cause the abdomen to become swollen and distended. In Keegan's case, even though he had a stoma at birth, his stoma was removed at nine months, and he continues to have the symptoms of abdominal distention because of his disease.

Vomiting: In more severe cases, the blockage can cause vomiting, which may be green or brownish in colour. Keegan has vomiting episodes, and thankfully, these are not very often. With Keegan's Hirschsprung's disease, monitoring his food intake and output is essential. If Keegan has not had a bowel movement for a day or two, one way his system can relieve itself is for him to vomit the food out of his system. Keegan does not like to vomit; he struggles with it, and I become apprehensive that he will choke because of his reluctance to vomit the food out of his body.

Delayed Growth: Chronic issues with feeding and digestion can cause poor weight gain and growth in affected infants. Keegan certainly had problems with feeding in the first few days of his life; however, he mastered the art of sucking his bottle and never looked back. He had no issues with weight gain or growth in infancy and continued to gain and grow as the years went on.

Diagnosing Hirschsprung's disease often involves a combination of medical history, physical examination, and diagnostic tests. One of the essential diagnostic tools is a contrast enema or a rectal biopsy. In a rectal biopsy, a small piece of tissue is removed from the affected colon area to confirm the absence of ganglion cells.

When Keegan was younger, I needed to monitor his stool movements, and I do so today. When Keegan was younger, and he seemed to be in distress or constipated, I would use an enema to clear his bowel so that he could feel the relief of his symptoms. As a new parent, I was very cautious because I did not want to harm my baby. The doctors and nurses at the doctor's offices and in the hospital offered me training and suggested how I could insert the enema for Keegan to release his pain. This I did, and sometimes I felt like a nurse and wondered if I should apply to nursing school.

Keegan's treatment for Hirschsprung's disease involved surgery to remove the segment of his colon lacking ganglion cells. This procedure is known as a pull-through operation, and the remaining healthy part of the colon is connected to the rectum. The extent of the surgery depends on the individual case and the length of the colon affected. Following surgery, most children, including Keegan, experience significant improvement in their ability to pass stool after doctors create a stoma for a child who has Hirschsprung's disease.

Creating a stoma in a child with Hirschsprung's disease involves a surgical procedure designed to alleviate the blockage and restore normal bowel function associated with this condition. This intricate process entails forming an opening in the abdominal wall through which a segment of the intestine is brought to the surface, facilitating the passage of stool.

PREOPERATIVE PREPARATION

Before the surgery, the medical team meticulously assess the child's overall health. This comprehensive evaluation encompasses blood tests, imaging studies such as X-rays or contrast enemas, and an examination to gauge the extent of the affected colon segment. The child's medical history, allergies, and specific considerations are thoroughly reviewed, ensuring a tailored and well-informed approach to the upcoming procedure.

Anesthesia:

The surgery is performed under general anesthesia to ensure that the child remains wholly asleep and pain-free throughout the procedure.

Incision:

The surgeon makes an incision in the abdominal wall. The location of the incision may vary depending on the case's specific circumstances. Still, it is typically made in the lower abdomen.

Exposing the Affected Segment:

After the incision, the surgeon gently exposes the affected segment of the colon, which lacks ganglion cells, and the healthy portion of the colon adjacent to it.

Creating the Stoma:

The healthy portion of the colon is brought out through the abdominal wall to form the stoma. The end of the colon is stitched to the skin, creating an opening in the abdomen. This stoma allows stool to bypass the affected segment of the colon, effectively relieving the obstruction.

Securing the Stoma:

The stoma is secured in place, and a unique bag, known as an ostomy bag, is fitted over the stoma to collect stool. The colostomy bag is designed to be quickly emptied and replaced as needed.

Closure:

The surgeon then closes the incision in the abdominal wall with stitches or surgical staples.

RECOVERY AND POSTOPERATIVE CARE

After the procedure, the child is carefully monitored in the recovery room. The medical team provides guidance on stoma care and how to manage the ostomy bag. Postoperative care includes pain management, monitoring for any signs of infection, and ensuring that the stoma is functioning properly.

Creating a stoma in a child with Hirschsprung's disease is a crucial step in managing the condition, as it allows for the bypass of the non-functioning portion of the colon, ultimately improving bowel function and the child's overall health. The surgical team works closely with the child's family to ensure they are well-informed about stoma care and any necessary follow-up appointments.

THE JOURNEY AHEAD

There was no roadmap for us in this unfamiliar terrain. Our primary focus was on Keegan's low muscle tone, which required constant physiotherapy. Our journey began with his feeding. His enlarged tongue made it challenging, and we needed to figure out how to help him eat. Then, we had to ensure he could digest the food properly, given that all his waste was diverted through a colostomy bag.

Keegan's ostomy bag became an integral part of his daily life. It allowed him to excrete waste through a stoma on his abdomen, creating a unique caregiving experience. Cleaning and changing the ostomy bag became a routine, much like changing diapers, but with the bag attached to his tummy.

For the first nine months of Keegan's life, I never changed a typical diaper. Instead, I managed his colostomy bag, a testament to the adaptability and strength that parents of children with special needs develop.

KATHLEEN'S GUIDE TO SUPPORTING KEEGAN'S NEEDS

Embarking on parenting a child with special needs requires navigating various tasks. Here is an overview of the steps I took to support Keegan:

UNDERSTANDING SPECIAL NEEDS

The first crucial step is to delve into understanding the specific condition or disability that Keegan faces. Whether it's intellectual disabilities, physical challenges, sensory impairments, or developmental disorders, gaining insight into the nuances of their unique needs is paramount. This knowledge forms the foundation for providing practical support.

SUPPORT NETWORK

Building a robust support network is essential. Connect with healthcare professionals, therapists, teachers, and fellow parents who have experience with children facing similar special needs. Engaging with support groups can provide invaluable insights and a sense of community. This network became a source of strength and shared wisdom, fostering a supportive environment for Keegan and me on this journey.

FEEDING

Catering to the unique dietary requirements or eating challenges of children with special needs demands specialised attention. Seek advice from a pediatrician or a nutritionist who can offer insights into addressing these issues. They are well-equipped to provide guidance on suitable diets and feeding techniques tailored to your child's specific needs.

CHANGING AND PERSONAL CARE

Adapting the approach to modifying and caring for your child is crucial. Consider incorporating specialised equipment such as adaptive changing tables or assistive devices to facilitate a more comfortable and efficient care routine.

MEDICAL NEEDS

Many children with special needs have ongoing medical requirements. Collaborate closely with their healthcare team to navigate the intricacies of managing these needs. This may involve discussions about medication administration, scheduling regular check-ups, and developing strategies for handling acute medical issues as they arise.

CHANGING DRESSINGS

For children requiring dressings or wound care, it's imperative to learn proper techniques from healthcare professionals. Ensuring their comfort and safety during these procedures is paramount, and professional guidance will empower you to confidently address their specific needs.

OPERATIONS AND PROCEDURES

In some cases, surgical interventions may be necessary. Be well-informed about the procedures, potential risks, and post-operative care. Discuss your child's unique situation with the surgical team.

CONSTANT TESTING

Frequent medical tests may be necessary to monitor your child's condition. These can be challenging, but they are essential for proper care. Work closely with your healthcare team to schedule and manage these tests.

PHYSIOTHERAPY AND THERAPY SERVICES

Many children with special needs benefit from physical, occupational, or speech therapy. These therapies can help improve your child's functioning and quality of life. Attend these sessions regularly and consider home exercises as well.

TOY LIBRARY AND ADAPTIVE PLAY

Explore resources like toy libraries and organisations that offer adaptive toys and equipment tailored to children with special needs. These can help with your child's development and enjoyment.

PATIENCE AND SELF-CARE

Parenting a child with special needs can be emotionally and physically challenging. Remember to take care of yourself. Seek respite care when needed, and ask for help from family and friends.

ADVOCACY AND LEGAL RIGHTS

Familiarise yourself with the legal rights and entitlements for children with special needs, including educational services, accommodations, and support under relevant laws like the Individuals with Disabilities Education Act in Australia.

FINANCIAL PLANNING

Special needs can be financially burdensome. Investigate available financial assistance, grants, and insurance options to help cover expenses related to your child's condition.

LONG-TERM PLANNING

Think about the future and what will happen when your child becomes an adult. Create a long-term plan that addresses housing, employment, and support services.

Remember that each child is unique, and their needs may evolve over time. Continuously communicate with healthcare professionals and support networks to adapt your parenting approach to best serve your child's well-being and development. Patience, love, and advocacy are essential throughout this journey.

In the next section, we'll explore how to navigate the complex world of medical care for your child with special needs. There is no one-size-fits-all solution, but with the proper knowledge and support, you can provide your child with the best care and opportunities for a fulfilling life.

CHAPTER 4

Engaging Therapies Early

In this chapter, I share my understanding of engaging Keegan in early therapies to help him grow and track his ongoing physical health and his emotional ability to manage tasks and learn new milestones. While there is no one-size-fits-all for a child with special needs, I believed it was crucial for me as Keegan's mum to set him up on the right path of his life with support to help him grow and continue to tailor his support to his unique needs.

SPEECH THERAPY

The beginning of Keegan's therapeutic journey was exciting for me and challenging for him. As Keegan grew older, he also developed a temper. We later learned it was due to his frustration at being unable to communicate effectively and share his wants and wishes. With the introduction of a speech therapist, Keegan could sit and follow instructions with his therapist and learn new words. Watching him try his best, I knew he would try again and learn to communicate with me.

One of the main words I wanted Keegan to learn was to call me mum, and his late dad also wanted to hear him call him dad. Although this was our wish, we were delighted when Keegan could say mum and dad. It is a small milestone he was so proud to achieve, and he knew when he said mum or dad, we would immediately respond.

Keegan benefited from his speech therapy sessions; I could see he could listen and express his feelings. His confidence increased, and he quickly learned the word 'no' when he did not want to follow guidance from me or his late dad. Keegan developed early language skills for his age from his speech therapy sessions. Although his speech was not fluent compared to a child without special needs, he did very well in not giving up. He continued practising his speech in the car while watching television or when he listened to the words I read.

OCCUPATIONAL THERAPY

Taking Keegan to his occupational therapist allowed me to learn new skills to continue his exercises and training at home. Because

Keegan had low muscle tone, his legs were weak, and he found it difficult and frustrating to stand up and get to where he needed to be. Keegan crawled when he was a year old and walked when he was two. Walking at two years old was an excellent achievement for Keegan, and I was satisfied that his early occupational therapies gave him a perfect start to sitting, crawling, and walking confidently.

Keegan continued to have occupational therapy throughout the different stages of his life. I taught him how to use the toilet independently through his occupational therapy sessions. How to make himself a sandwich, cut bread, and eat with a knife and fork. While we take some of these tasks for granted, for Keegan, it was skills he needed to develop and be taught how to hold the utensils and feed himself.

Keegan's occupational therapy sessions today occur in our home. Tim has become a guiding light in teaching him how to use the washing machine, pack and unpack the dishwasher, and his ongoing personal care routine.

One of the great things about Keegan is that he is willing to try, and he has this pleased look on his face when he knows he completed a task and can do it without being prompted. Keegan continues to challenge me, and I am sure it goes without saying that most children challenge their parents. Yet, they will do it for their teacher, speech, and occupational therapist.

SWIMMING

Keegan loves water and enjoys going to the swimming pool. Our house in Randburg had a swimming pool, and we moved to this house when Keegan was seven years old. I arranged for Keegan and his brother Bradlee to go for swimming lessons. Taking them to swimming lessons allowed me to watch their ability to learn water safety and swim and enjoy swimming in the pool at home.

Bradlee became a very confident swimmer. Keegan, on the other hand, still loves to swim his way. He learned to kick his legs and straighten his body in the pool; however, he never forgot about opening his eyes in the water. I am not sure where he learned to do this; however, it may be from the times he wore swimming goggles during his swimming lessons so he could keep his eyes open. Even today, Keegan can stay in the water for as long as he chooses and not get tired of swimming his way.

Swimming lessons for Bradlee and Keegan taught them water safety and how to keep themselves safe in the water. Even though Keegan understands water safety, he is never on his own while swimming.

BIKE WITH NO PEDDLES

Keegan's legs and balance improved, so he learned to ride his two-wheel bike. His bike had a handlebar, two wheels, and no peddles. This meant Keegan had to use his legs to push himself on his motorcycle. And so he did. Keegan was determined to get on his bike and learn to push himself, and was very proud when he could do it all alone. While Keegan was riding his bike like an expert, his brother Bradlee also had a bike with no peddles, and they learned to race each other on the side of the house.

It was early on a Saturday morning. Keegan and Bradlee decided to ride their bikes around the house, and I could hear them talking and laughing together. Suddenly, there was silence, and I could not see them from the kitchen or the side window that overlooked our driveway. I saw an open front gate and no sight of the boys. I yelled out to my late husband and asked him if the boys were with him in the garage, and he said no. I ran down the driveway, and all I could see was Keegan and Bradlee riding their bikes in the middle of the road and using their little feet to run away from home.

I was so shocked at what they both did and by this time, they were about 300 metres from home. As I watched for traffic, they saw me and thought it was a game, and I was chasing them, so they pushed themselves faster. I was terrified, and I finally caught up with them, held their hands, and steered them to the footpath.

Our road did not have a concrete footpath. However, there was grass, and I encouraged Keegan and Bradlee to ride their bikes on the grass. Keegan was unhappy because he found it difficult to push himself on the grass footpath and I eventually carried the bikes, made them hold hands, and walked home.

PHYSICAL THERAPY

Keegan attended daycare when he was three years old. At daycare, he learned daily exercises with the other children in his group. He learnt quickly, and one skill he picked up from his physical therapy sessions was learning to run in races at daycare and eventually at school and becoming a Special Olympics athlete.

Keegan enjoyed going to Special Olympics training and events. His group of friends shared common interests in rugby, swimming and athletics. He enjoyed the plane rides to different parts of the country to compete in athletic events. He was very proud of himself when he received his gold, silver, and bronze medals.

Enrolling Keegan in physical therapeutic exercises encouraged him to run in athletic competitions and be part of the athletics team.

PUSH CART

To encourage Keegan to walk, his occupational therapist suggested we buy a wooden cart at the local toy store. His therapist suggested we remove the wooden blocks and put 2 bricks in the pushcart. Following her instructions, we did just that and encouraged Keegan to hold the handlebar and push the cart.

At first, he was very apprehensive because the cart moved, and as we drove the cart slowly, he learned he needed to use his arms to push the cart's weight so it could move. When the cart moved, he did not move his legs to be closer to the cart. He let it go and sat on the ground.

Keegan continued to try to push his cart daily until one day he learned how to move his feet and be in sync with the cart when it moved. I was so excited for him, and although he tried, he still needed encouragement and support to remind him he could do it.

Keegan continued to push his cart, and he learned to load it with the toys he wanted in the cart. He found the pushing to be fun, and one day, he eventually let the cart go and learnt to walk on his own. Even though he learned to walk unaided, he still played with his cart and loaded sand, food, toys, and anything he could find in his cart. Purchasing the cart when Keegan was much younger gave him the time to learn and become confident at walking independently.

CHAPTER 5

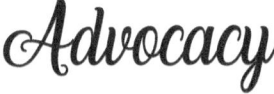

I grew up with a strong sense of social justice. When my child was born with a disability, I didn't expect it would prompt me to switch careers. I became a social worker to better understand how he accessed services and support and to ensure he received the best care from the right people.

Caring for Keegan has taught me valuable lessons.

HERE ARE 10 STEPS I'VE LEARNED

EDUCATE ME

Learning about Keegan's disability and related challenges was crucial for adequate care. I believe it is essential to understand my child's disability, as I talked about earlier. I needed to learn about the different types of disabilities and the challenges my child, Keegan, might face as he grows up. I needed to understand the rights of individuals with disabilities and stay informed of the laws and regulations in three countries.

LISTEN AND LEARN

I learnt to listen and learn from and for Keegan. He gave me signals and words and showed me what he wanted when he wanted and did not want something, such as food, a game or visiting a friend or family member. I encouraged him to speak up and say what he liked and disliked so I could learn from him. Learning from Keegan was not the only adjustment I needed to make. I also needed to listen to the doctor's feedback on how I could support Keegan and learn from the experiences. In supporting or advocating for Keegan, as he grew older, I needed to involve him in his decision-making processes.

PROMOTE INCLUSIVITY

While the world was making changes to be more inclusive for children with disabilities in places like doctor's offices, hospitals, and schools, there were still challenges. Some areas didn't have facilities for disabled people. Even though this is happening less often now, I always remember that Keegan has special needs. It's beneficial for him and makes things less stressful for me when I advocate for services that include him in different environments.

RAISE AWARENESS

In my daily life, at work and during travel, I subtly raise awareness, especially when services aren't suitable for Keegan. Once, during a family visit to warm baths in New Zealand, the changing area had facilities for people with disabilities. However, since Keegan is male, he couldn't enter the female change room with me, and I couldn't go into the male change room with him. After waiting in line and seeing Keegan shivering, I noticed the men's change room had no line. Holding Keegan's hand, we entered the male change room, used the disability facility, and left with smiles. Meanwhile, the line for the women's change room kept growing. I later spoke with the establishment's owner, who acknowledged the challenges faced by disabled individuals and agreed with my approach to address the situation for Keegan and me.

COLLABORATE WITH DISABILITY AGENCIES

Working closely with disability agencies helps build a support network and ensures Keegan receives the necessary assistance. To ensure Keegan received the required support from disability agencies, I felt it was crucial to familiarise myself with the day program, his school, teachers, and the school's operation. Attending school events, functions, and parent discussions became the best way to understand support systems and hear from parents and professionals in the disability system. Keegan's teachers knew me as 'Keegan's Mum', a title I'm still known by among his friends. In the disability world, it's more common for people to remember you as the child's parent rather than by your name. I find it heartwarming to be called Keegan's Mum because it reflects the connections I've built while getting to know the essential individuals who support Keegan daily. Collaborative efforts often have a more significant impact.

NAVIGATE LEGAL RIGHTS

Understanding the legal rights and protections of individuals with disabilities is essential to secure assistance. As a parent of a child with a disability, I had to understand the legal rights and protections for individuals with disabilities. When we moved to New Zealand, Keegan, being a permanent resident, couldn't receive financial assistance because his disability didn't originate in New Zealand or Australia. While it seems discriminatory, the current country of residence provides financial support. However, he doesn't qualify for a disability pension. Instead, he qualifies for a special benefit, which requires an ongoing effort from him and me. Keegan has to consistently prove his inability to work to maintain financial support. Our ongoing goal is to work towards him receiving forty hours of support so he can eventually be employed and earn financial rewards.

BUILD STRONG COMMUNICATION SKILLS

Developing practical communication skills helps express Keegan's needs and coordinates support from schools, doctors, and agencies. Living in three countries with Keegan over the years, I had to develop strong communication skills as his mom. It was important to express his concerns, articulate what he needed from conversations, and outline how schools, doctors, or social service agencies could support him. Given my inquisitive nature, I often delved into the details of Keegan's needs, requesting reports to stay updated on assessment outcomes and recommended treatments. Emailing doctors' offices, schools, or agencies proved effective. It created a documented trail of our discussions, ensuring accountability for the commitments made to support Keegan.

ENGAGE WITH DECISION-MAKERS

Working closely with disability agencies helps build a support network and ensures Keegan receives the necessary assistance. Connect with policymakers, legislators, and other decision-makers to advocate for changes that improve the lives of individuals with disabilities. Participate in public forums, write letters, and attend meetings to voice your concerns.

BE YOUR CHILD'S ADVOCATE

Being a persistent advocate ensures Keegan receives the support he needs, whether at school, in healthcare, or elsewhere. Encourage individuals with disabilities to advocate for themselves. Provide them the tools and knowledge to express their needs and preferences independently.

STAY PERSISTENT

Stay Inquisitive. Asking questions and checking details ensures a clear understanding of Keegan's requirements, assessments, and recommended treatments. Advocacy often requires persistence. Be prepared to navigate challenges, setbacks, and bureaucracy. Continue to advocate for positive change over the long term. Remember, effective advocacy is a continuous process that involves ongoing education, collaboration, and a commitment to promoting equality and inclusion.

CHAPTER 6

Education

Growing up, I recognised the importance of education for everyone. When you have a child with a disability, the landscape of education changes. It requires thinking creatively because the education system for children without disabilities differs. I had to confront the reality that specific daycare centres and schools might not accept Keegan because of a lack of disability inclusivity; but I did not give up.

Keegan always had many family and friends around him, and he quickly learned from everyone. When he was three months old, I returned to work, so my mother-in-law, Maureen, kindly cared for him from three months to one year. Keegan stayed with her during the week, and on Fridays, we picked him up to spend the weekend together. It was a tough choice, but it helped us financially.

At one year old, we hired a full-time nanny for Keegan, but we faced challenges as some nannies were scared of his disability. When he turned three, I tried enrolling him in a local daycare, but they weren't equipped for children with disabilities. Undeterred, I explored other options, speaking with people in the education and disability sectors and our community.

I met Mercy, a mum with a son attending a school for children with disabilities in Lenasia. Mercy shared the contact information, and after discussions and visits, Keegan was accepted into their daycare program. Mavis, a wonderful nanny, took care of him. She prepared his breakfast, packed his bag, and walked him to the school bus outside our home. The Jiswa School for Children with Disabilities provided transportation, making it convenient for us.

Keegan would happily hop on the bus, waving his little hand, and off he went to daycare. When he returned home, he was joyful, and this routine continued until we moved to a different suburb.

UNDERSTANDING THE BARRIERS TO INCLUSIVE EDUCATION

Being a parent of a child with a disability, I found the journey through the educational system quite challenging. I had never experienced it before and had to learn where Keegan could and could not attend school. In 1996, after some time, my late husband and I agreed to sell our house in Ennerdale and move sixty-five kilometres away to a new suburb closer to the city and closer to his work. Selling our home was easy; however, we needed to consider where Keegan would go to school. Keegan was seven years old, and the search for a new school in a new suburb was less stressful than before. I had had the experience of finding him a daycare centre, and now this was him going to school.

After several phone calls, completing application forms and attending interviews, Keegan was offered a spot in a Montessori School in Randburg. What a relief. Keegan could go to school, make friends, and learn. This school was for disabled children from five to seventeen years old, and it was a relief that Keegan could stay there until he turned seventeen. Keegan's school was on my way to work, and we would drive to school in the morning, singing songs and listening to the top hits on the radio. I found it a perfect arrangement, close to home and work, and I could drop off and pick up Keegan from school and his younger brother Bradlee from daycare.

NAVIGATING DISABILITY EDUCATION IN A NEW COUNTRY

In the year 1997, Keegan, Bradlee and I said goodbye to my late husband, who died suddenly. His death came as a huge shock, and I made a heartbreaking decision to move my children from South Africa to New Zealand. In 1999, Keegan, Bradlee and I got on an Australian Qantas Aircraft and said goodbye to our motherland. We arrived, spent two weeks holiday with my sisters in Sydney, Australia and moved to New Zealand at the end of July 1999. This was the mark of our new journey to the unknown for the children because I had visited New Zealand in 1998 to spend time with my sister and cousins and to find time to recuperate after my husband's premature death.

Arriving in New Zealand gave us a new start and a new plan to move forward with our lives without my late husband and for the children, their beloved dad. I followed the same method I used previously to find Keegan a school. By this time, Keegan was ten years old, and Bradlee was five. Lucky for me, my sister Karen taught at a local primary school, so she took Bradlee along to school, registered him in kindy and off he went to school.

With Keegan, I phoned the leading disability schools. I was given an interview for him at Mt Richmond Special School in Otahuhu. Joining the Mt Richmond school community was a blessing. Keegan was enrolled in an inclusive school with a class designed for children with special needs. He was not separated from the school. He had access to the school and attended Manurewa East School until he completed year six.

Keegan was picked up at home in the morning, transported to school, and then to his after-school program. He waited with his brother Bradlee for me to pick them up after work. Later on, I arranged for Keegan and Bradlee to attend before and after school care, and they quickly changed their routine of me dropping them off and picking them up in the afternoon. At the before and after school program, Keegan was treated no differently than the other children in the club. If he did not follow the rules, I would receive a letter from the supervisor, which would be true for Bradlee. My boys continued in the before and after school program until my late mum came to live in New Zealand.

When my late mum, Granny, came to live with us, everything changed again. We learnt new routines; Keegan could hop on the disability transport, and Bradlee took the bus to and from his school. Both boys quickly learnt their new routines. My routine changed because there was no longer drop off and pick up in the mornings and afternoons, and this gave me a little time to spend by myself before I hopped on the bus to the city for work.

When Keegan finished year six at his primary school, he attended Papatoetoe Intermediate School, which had special needs classes attached to the school. Here, he made friends and went to school with most of his friends from primary school. Keegan enjoyed going to school because it was fun for him. He learned cooking, sport, horticulture, and music. He loved attending school camps, playing rugby, and participating in the Special Olympics, where he took part in shotput and athletics.

Bradlee and I followed Keegan around the country with his activities. We enjoyed making friends with the parents and the children from his school and the Special Olympics teams. One year, Keegan was chosen to represent his school in the Special Olympics in Christchurch, New Zealand. Bradlee and I followed the group and attended the week-long event with a little sightseeing. It was a week of fun, laughter, and admiration for people with disabilities who played sports and participated in events that made them happy.

We continued to navigate the education system in New Zealand until Keegan left school at eighteen. Keegan could no longer attend Mt Richmond School, and the future planning teachers arranged meetings for us to meet with them and community agencies to support Keegan when he left school. When Keegan left school, he attended a day program close to our home, where he needed to make new friends and adjust to his daily routine and the schedule he chose to continue his learning needs. Keegan decided to do cooking, mowing lawns, going for walks, swimming, and painting.

He wanted to be part of a community and found his place in the day program.

Historically, people with disabilities were institutionalised or segregated from their communities. I am so grateful I had the common sense to not take my doctor's advice because Keegan has led me on a path of self-discovery, and in most cases, I had to learn from his disability and follow him where he went to ensure that his educational needs were met.

And another country move was planned. In 2011, it was time to pack up and move across the ditch to Sydney, Australia. Not again, I thought. However, it was time to unsettle the family and re-settle them in a new land for the final time. I hope it is. Moving to Australia was a mammoth task. This time, it was Keegan, Bradlee, my late mum (Granny) and me. The four of us embarked on a new journey to live closer to family and friends in the sunny state of New South Wales. Selling our home in Auckland, New Zealand, was quick, and I didn't have time to plan long goodbyes. I needed to pack my home again into a container, and off we flew to Sydney.

Setting up a home in Sydney's Western Suburbs gave me time to find Keegan a daily community program and work for me. Keegan was fortunate to receive block funding after a year at home in a community agency where he went daily. Knowing that Keegan was settled, Bradlee attended TAFE in Blacktown and embarked on a journey to find his passion and what he wanted to do with his time and career. I worked for a non-government agency. After a year, I left that organisation to move to a more prominent non-government agency.

A year after we arrived in Australia, the Australian government changed how people were funded to support their disability. Block funding, as they called it in 2011, was no longer how non-government agencies were funded. The funding model meant that each disabled person would be supported according to their needs and goals. This was a massive change for me, as well as for Keegan. With the new funding model, Keegan could purchase the support he needed to be active in his community and do what he wanted to do with his time.

Having a new National Disability Insurance Scheme (NDIS) Plan, Keegan could purchase services from Afford, a non-government agency in Western Sydney, Blacktown. He continues attending the day program designed for his needs. Keegan has many friends at his day program and chooses the activities he wishes to do daily. Keegan enjoys bowling, cooking, going to pub lunch, swimming, athletics and exercising with his peers in the park. Keegan has done sailing, travel training, and loved gardening; however, he chooses not to work in the garden.

I looked at all the practical strategies for parents, educators, and policymakers in educating Keegan. I made decisions based on Keegan's best interests. Advocating for Keegan was a daily routine, and yes, you need to navigate the bureaucratic maze and work towards making education fun and workable for your child, as I did for Keegan. Disability education rights for people have evolved over the years. It is instrumental that your child goes to school to be part of a wider community.

I've picked up some valuable education tips for children and young adults with disabilities:

- Ensure children with disabilities get a good education in a supportive learning setting.
- Design learning materials and activities accessible to all students, including those with disabilities.

- Allow students to learn and access information in a way that suits their needs best.
- All students, including those with disabilities, should have an Individualised Education Plan (IEP) tailored to meet their educational needs.
- Keep up the collaboration and communication between teachers, parents, and specialists to ensure everyone works together for the student's success.

CHAPTER 7

Building a Support Network

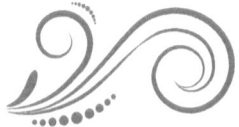

I have four sisters and two brothers, forming a tribe. Expanding my support network was a way to enlarge my family circle. Initially, I didn't realise how big my tribe had become. Now, after living in three countries, I am grateful that my tribe extends beyond the borders of Australia.

With any child, irrespective of whether a child has or has no special needs, parents take the time to build a network when their child is born. This network grows and grows; sometimes, people fall off your network, and you pick up new people. I learnt this after moving to different countries. In South Africa, I had a solid, stable support network. I could call upon any family member to help me care for Keegan and Bradlee. There was no shortage of friends and family to help when needed. I also had a nanny for the children, which was a huge help, and a family who always lived close by and were willing to have the kids over for the day or night.

As a young single parent, I found the responsibilities and stress more daunting. Now, I needed to make decisions on my own and hope they were the right decisions for both my children. One way of relieving my stress was to build a support network, which I found very helpful. The support network or support systems were outside of my family circle. They were crucial for my emotional well-being, sharing knowledge, and learning to manage the challenges of raising one child with special needs and one without a disability.

Both my children required hospitalisation at different times in their lives. When Bradlee was three years old, he was hospitalised for asthma. Luckily, our nanny lived with us, and she could take care of Keegan while I stayed in the hospital with Bradlee until he was discharged from care. Support systems are needed when children become unwell, especially if you are a single parent; juggling time and energy on each child can be daunting. The good thing about Bradlee's hospitalisation was that he was placed in an oxygen tent, and we slept there for two nights. I had the best sleep ever in the oxygen tent and he left the hospital as energetic as ever. I would not have been able to stay with Bradlee in the hospital had I had no support system in place to help me help him through his illness and support his recovery.

The importance of organising a support system as a parent of a child with special needs cannot be overstated. Parenting a child with special needs is a complex and demanding role that can lead to feelings of isolation, stress, and burnout. Connecting with friends, family, and outside family support and going through similar experiences can provide a sense of belonging and understanding that can be difficult to find elsewhere. I always felt that support networks offer a safe space to share my feelings, frustrations and successes of parenting my two boys.

Some ways to build a support network and maintain my tribe:

MY FAMILY

I relied on my family and friends to help me parent my sons Keegan and Bradlee. My mother-in-law cared for Keegan for three months until he turned one and continued caring for him when he was at her home.

When Keegan was four months old, my cousin Memory, who lived in Johannesburg near me, travelled to Durban to visit family. She asked if she could take Keegan with her for a holiday. I agreed, and he saw his aunties, uncles, and grandmother in Durban. I taught Memory how to change Keegan's colostomy bag, and she showed my late mum and my sisters. He had a wonderful holiday, and I had a break.

After my husband died, I planned a trip to visit my sisters in New Zealand and Australia. I prepared for the visit and asked my late mum to care for Keegan and Bradlee while I was away. My late mum supported me on the trip and asked me to bring the children to Durban to spend time with their cousins there. I quickly booked the plane tickets for Keegan, Bradlee and the nanny and off they went on a plane ride to Durban for a month to stay with their granny. I enjoyed the overseas respite, learnt how to relax and recuperate, and felt fresh returning home to the children. I missed them, though.

Reducing my isolation was also one way to build and maintain relationships.

My friend Beryl lived close to me and always wanted us at her place. And she visited me regularly, and we spoke on the phone most days.

My dear friends Evangeline (Venge), Debbie, and Penny lived close to me and supported me immensely. I was able to pack my children and spend the day with them, be fed, and sometimes Venge made new clothing outfits for me, and off home I went.

My friends and family provided me with a listening ear. They always made me feel welcome and part of their family or gave me a helping hand when I needed it most.

Support systems don't only involve family and friends:

SEEK OUT SUPPORT GROUPS

There are many support groups for parents of children with disabilities. These support groups offer valuable resources, and talking to parents facing similar, if not the same, challenges can make the session at the group rewarding. Sometimes, I felt I was doing it tough. Yet, some parents were finding it more challenging than me, with varying degrees of disability and support needed.

Doctor's rooms became a social point for me at one time. I was visiting the doctors so regularly, like clockwork. Little did I know that doctors, nurses, and specialists would become part of my social calendar because you need to be organised, have a great plan to keep appointments, and be part of the medical environment more times than I could have imagined.

Hospital admissions were also an excellent time to talk to parents whose children needed surgery, and it gave me time to interact with adults and talk about Keegan. If I chose not to speak on a particular day, I would sleep in the hospital chair. However, most times, it is better to talk to other parents because we all have the same fears and worries when our children are admitted to the hospital.

PRACTICAL ASSISTANCE. This support can be arranged anytime, including respite care, assistance with daily living, and transport.

Respite Care is one way for me, and I imagine for parents of children with a disability to take time out for myself or yourself. I have respite care for Keegan, where he goes into a group home managed by a non-government agency and stays there for up to two to four nights or longer if needed. Last year, I needed to travel to South Africa, and Keegan stayed at his respite home for twenty-six nights. He missed his room and his bed and was very happy to see me when he came home.

Keegan has assistance with his daily living, and a community of support workers were arranged to help him with his personal care and preparing his afternoon snack while I was at work. Keegan says he is happy with this arrangement and spends time with the support worker to assist him with his needs.

Keegan and I have a choice when it comes to his transportation. His NDIS plan includes funding for him to be taken to and from his daily program. Currently, Keegan is being transported to and from his program. He likes the music in the van and gets to travel with his friends, getting picked up in the morning and dropped off at home in the afternoon.

Therapists and Counselors: professional support can be incredibly beneficial, both for the child and the parents. Therapists and counsellors can offer guidance, coping strategies, and a safe space to process emotions. Utilise professional resources: consult with your child's healthcare providers and therapists to inquire about support groups or resources they recommend. Explore government and community-based organisations that offer support services for special needs families. Seek professional mental health support when necessary.

ALLIED HEALTH PROFESSIONALS

Occupational Therapist – ongoing support
Speech Therapist – ongoing support
Physiotherapy – supports when needed
Personal Trainer – in the process of setting this up

Medical Specialists

General Practitioner
Urologist
Neurologist
Dermatologist
Optometrist

Dentist
Dietitian – in the process of setting this up
Podiatrist

Grooming

Barber – he loves cutting his hair
Shaving – I had to learn this, and Keegan finds this task very daunting

Clothing

He can choose his own clothing and dress himself (when he is in the mood to do it)

ONLINE COMMUNITIES

I found several online platforms for parents and social media groups dedicated to special needs parents. Sometimes, talking to people in a chat group experiencing the same challenges is more manageable than being alone. Social media groups are a great support.

UTILISE COMMUNITY RESOURCES

Investigate local resources such as respite care, special education services, and organisations that assist families with special needs children:

- Connect with other parents- seek out local or online support groups and forums specifically designed for parents of special needs children. These communities provide a wealth of shared experiences and advice. Attend local events, workshops, or seminars on special needs parenting to meet others facing similar challenges.

- Community Resources and Support Groups- local Support Groups: many communities have local support groups that meet regularly. These groups can be a great way to connect with parents facing similar challenges. Look for information about these groups at community centres, schools, or through healthcare providers.
- Non-Profit Organisations- numerous non-profit organisations are dedicated to helping families with special needs children. They often provide resources, guidance, and access to support networks.

SELF-CARE

Foster Self-Care - remember that taking care of yourself is just as important. A well-rested and emotionally balanced parent is better equipped to care for their child. Caring for a child with special needs can be emotionally taxing. Support from friends, family, and fellow parents provides a safe space to share feelings, vent frustrations, and find empathy. Schedule regular breaks and ensure you have time for self-care and relaxation.

Building a support network may require effort and time, but the benefits are immeasurable. It's an investment in your well-being and the well-being of your child. By connecting with others who understand your journey, you can find strength, resilience, and a community that will support you through the challenges and joys of special needs parenting.

Building a Support Network

Raising a child with special needs can be a rewarding but challenging journey. Parents and caregivers often navigate a complex world of medical, educational, and emotional needs. In these circumstances, having a solid support network is crucial for maintaining physical and emotional well-being.

CHAPTER 8

Managing The Emotional Rollercoaster

I wasn't aware of the emotional challenges that come with parenting a special needs child. In this chapter, I explore the challenges I needed to face and how I overcame them. The right strategies and support network got me through my parenting journey. Although it looked smooth on the outside, sometimes, there were times when I needed to bring the rollercoaster to a halt.

Facing uncertainty for your child can be daunting. I grappled with the fate of Keegan's future, his development and the challenges he may meet with having a disability. I mentally prepared his lifespan and imagined how his life would be if I was not around to care for him. I was uncertain of his medical condition and how he would cope with Hirschbrungs disease, epilepsy, and asthma. Every day is new, and while the uncertainty fades as the years go on, having a sound support system and a robust plan for Keegan gives me peace of mind.

Experiencing grief and loss for a child's development, relationship, education, health, and well-being is unexpected. You share the loss of your child, yet your child is living and going about their day-to-day stuff. The loss is more around Keegan not having a typical bowel system, not being able to breathe sometimes, and also at any time he could have a seizure. The loss on some days can be immense because he has lost out on so many experiences in his life due to his health and well-being. Grief is an emotion that creeps up on you. You may not know that you are actually grieving the loss of your child's relationships and the possibility of him not getting married or having children of his own. These are my realities, and sometimes it's easier to focus on the here and now than think too far into the future or dwell on what could have been, knowing full well it may never eventuate.

I sometimes found connecting with others who did not understand my situation challenging. I isolated myself from parent groups, online chat groups, and some of my robust support networks. Keeping myself safe from negative comments, especially on social media, was healthy. I found it very easy to disconnect myself from social media as it was not helpful for my health and well-being. When I saw the energy and the space for social media groups again, I rejoined with a different focus on what I needed from the group. If it did not support what I needed, I would gladly leave the area of communication and seek out different support.

Parenting Keegan sometimes contributed to high stress levels and, in some cases, burnout. I experienced high levels of anxiety after my husband died suddenly and realised I was solely responsible for raising Keegan and his brother Bradlee on my own. This thought was daunting, and I had no idea how I would manage raising two boys without their Dad. I worried or stressed about the children's health, education and safety. I needed to know where they were and how to contact them even now that they were adults.

Calculating the expenses for Keegan's medical care, therapy, and special education posed financial challenges, especially in his early life stages. When he moved to New Zealand, the local health system covered his medical needs and education. Although there was a copay for doctor visits, things changed when we arrived in Australia.

During our brief stay in Australia, Keegan had a seizure, and I had to rush to Newcastle from Sydney, where my sister had called an ambulance. At the hospital, concerns arose about Keegan's health, compounded by his lack of an Australian Medicare Card. Without this card, I was informed that I would be responsible for covering the substantial costs of his medical treatment.

In a moment of worry, a hospital administrator approached me and escorted me to the primary office. There, I learned that, as Keegan wasn't a permanent resident of Australia and lacked a Medicare Card, I needed to sign an agreement to pay his hospital bill before discharge. Despite the potential financial strain, I agreed without hesitation.

Shortly afterwards, a hospital employee inquired if I had applied for a Medicare Card. Confirming that I had, she informed me that if I had already applied, the hospital would waive the medical costs and contact Medicare for the necessary details. This was due to an agreement between Australia and New Zealand regarding medical care for New Zealand citizens.

Leaving the hospital, I felt relieved and grateful for the support and understanding of the personnel. The situation highlighted the importance of navigating healthcare systems in different countries and the significance of agreements that ease financial burdens for individuals needing medical care.

Advocating for Keegan extended beyond just medical situations, and at times, I found myself experiencing Advocacy Fatigue. The constant effort to set up systems, spending hours on the phone managing his services, and dealing with bureaucracy became overwhelming. There were moments when I just wished people would listen to my requests without complications or unnecessary changes.

Recently, when I needed to update Keegan's provider details, I faced a challenging battle that lasted for weeks. Feeling exhausted, I eventually gave up, realising that the proposed changes were not harming Keegan. The agency could handle any necessary adjustments themselves.

Following a call from the department, they requested Keegan to complete a nominee form, making me his nominee to act on his behalf. Despite my efforts, the process became more complicated. Even with Keegan's attempt to provide information, the government official couldn't identify him on their system.

Realising I needed a new strategy, I took a few days to step back and focus on other tasks. When I called the same office again, a different person answered and efficiently changed Keegan's profile on the government database in just a few seconds. This success left me both elated and grateful, even though Keegan couldn't understand why his mother had been making a fuss. This experience highlighted the persistence required in advocating for the needs of a special needs child and the importance of finding alternative approaches to navigate bureaucratic challenges.

Parenting Keegan with a disability and Bradlee with no disability was a constant balancing act. I knew that more time was given to Keegan or that he needed more attention than Bradlee. Bradlee was not shy in letting me know that my focus was totally on Keegan and was honest in sharing his feelings. Even though he shared how he felt, Bradlee understood his brother's disability and that Keegan needed more support than he did. Although Bradlee could understand the difference in my parenting, it did not take away the guilt of trying to balance my parenting style and time and focus on two children with totally different needs who needed my attention at other times in their lives.

I think it is every parent's fear when they think of their child's future. While some parents can plan their child's education, marriage, and potentially going on their OE – OE-overseas experience after year 12, parents of children with disabilities may have different fears. It is a fear for the future. Fear for the future is a valid fear for me. No one can say what will happen in the future. I had to make arrangements, because if I am no longer around who will care for Keegan and Bradlee? The Fear is also around the physical day-to-day care for Keegan, and although I don't dwell on this as much as I did before, it is undoubtedly at the back of my mind when I plan holiday trips, visit family interstate and when he goes off to respite. Another fear that may crop up occasionally is Keegan's health. What will this potentially look like as he ages? How will he tell me if he has a pain in his chest, leg, or arm? I can only see by his actions that there is something not right with him physically, which makes me ask him more questions, and this can lead to finding out an unknown injury or body ache unknown to him and me or those who care for him.

Caring for Keegan means I must bring my A-game to support him. I need to set the daily routine; in most cases, Keegan will go along with the planned day because he is used to the daily routine. Most days, he will ask the same questions; for instance, his one question is, "Staying home?", meaning can he stay home that day. My typical response will be, we cannot stay home today. Mum is going to work, and you go bowling, swimming, cooking, pub lunch and the park, depending on the day of the week and his planned activity at his program. If he sometimes becomes a bit ratty, I will try changing his focus from staying home to what he would like for breakfast. 99% of the time, it works. He knows our routine and the next steps for the day. He also has an afternoon routine: come home, shower, snack and do stuff he chooses to do before dinner.

While I was good at organising Keegan's schedule and ensuring everything ran smoothly, I realised I also had to figure out how to manage my feelings and well-being. It's essential to not just handle external tasks, but to also look after myself emotionally. When I felt I needed a holiday, I asked family and friends to care for Keegan and Bradlee when they were little. To have a break from my full-time caring role, Bradlee sometimes says, "Mum, you need to take a break. Go away for a few days, and I will look after Keegan". And so I did just that. It does not take long to twist my arm to go away for a few days or weeks. When my late Mum lived with me and helped me care for the boys, she was delighted when I went away, and I could travel more, have more frequent holidays, just rest, relax, and come home and start again. Now, it is just Keegan and me in the home. He has grown into a fine young man, he needs very little attention, and if I want to go away, I usually take him, or he stays with one of his aunties or goes to respite.

CHAPTER 9

Resilient Mum, Single Carer, Social Worker, And Ndis Registered Provider

In this chapter, I share the transformative journey that led me to embrace my resilience and embark on a path to becoming an NDIS Registered Provider. It was not easy. Juggling the roles of a devoted mother to Keegan, a full-time carer, and a Social Worker, I immersed myself in many challenges and responsibilities. However, realising my inherent resilience empowered me to navigate these complexities and make impactful decisions, including the pursuit of becoming a Registered Provider.

Resilience, the capacity to rebound from adversity, became evident as I faced the demands of motherhood, caregiving, and my professional role as a Social Worker. Maintaining a positive outlook, adapting to evolving circumstances, and crafting innovative solutions to surmount obstacles were markers of my resilience.

The pivotal choice to become an NDIS Registered Provider demanded careful consideration, and my resilience emerged as the catalyst for confidence in pursuing this opportunity. Recognising that this path would allow me to make a positive difference in the lives of individuals with disabilities and champion their independence fueled my determination. My story captures a personal triumph and a commitment to fostering independence and positive change in the lives of those within the disability community.

Resilient Mum, Single Carer, Social Worker, And Ndis Registered Provider

A VIEW OF MY TIMELINE

1989 - 26-year-old – son born with a disability

1994 - 31 years old – the second son born

1997 - 34 years old – husband dies suddenly

1999 – Emigrate to New Zealand

2003 – Career change from Financial Industry to Social Work

2010 – Diploma in Life Coaching NZ

2011 – Emigrate to Australia

2023 – Become NDIS Registered Provider

Despite being a mum to a child with a disability, I didn't let it stop me from pursuing my goals. In 2002, a significant change in my work hours posed a challenge. The demanding morning and afternoon pickups for my sons became unmanageable due to the new schedule. This not only affected our finances but also created stress. Making a courageous decision, I left my job in the financial industry, unsure of how I'd handle the mortgage and provide for my children. Fortunately, help came unexpectedly. A coworker named Sandy approached me, curious about why I was leaving. I explained the difficulties with the proposed hours and the impact on my stress levels, especially concerning picking up my boys from after-care on time. Little did I know that this challenging situation would eventually provide a solution.

Sandy handed me a paper with a phone number and said, "Call this number. You deserve a break." So, cautiously, I dialled the number, letting the lady know I was told to call. After making inquiries, I was invited for an interview. I gathered the needed documents and patiently waited. The interview went well, and I got approved for a parenting payment to help with my mortgage and support my children. I was in total shock; I didn't know about this service. I never thought I could have time with my kids, stay home, and have a regular life. Emigrating to a new country brought different opportunities. This was my chance not only to find another job and give back to my community, but also to take time for myself and rethink my life's next steps. So, I set out a plan for myself.

I saw a notice in the local newspaper and applied for a volunteer position at Victims Support. After completing the training, I found joy in the role. While there, I connected with volunteers studying to become Social Workers. Curious, I inquired about becoming a counsellor and soon realised that being a Social Worker was better for me. Going back to university wasn't initially part of my plan. Still, with the support of student loans, my children, and my family, I took the leap. In 2006, I successfully completed my Bachelor of Social Work.

Upon graduating from university, I applied for a permanent role at Victim Support, a non-government agency. In this position, I was responsible for recruiting and training volunteers. These volunteers were on standby to provide support to victims of various crimes, ranging from motor vehicle accidents, home invasions, burglaries, sudden deaths, suicides, homicides, and cases involving babies who died suddenly at home. I worked to support women and children affected by domestic violence. This role significantly fortified my career, and the invaluable training I received played a crucial role in my professional development.

While my work at Victim Support was crucial for my professional growth, it also played a key role in navigating the right help and support for my son, Keegan. Supporting individuals in my community allowed me to extend that knowledge to meet Keegan's needs, leveraging my relationships with community agencies in my area and beyond. As life in New Zealand settled, my late Mum celebrated her eightieth birthday, and my family came to join the celebration. During a late-night conversation with my sister Joan, she suggested, "Why don't you and Karen move to Australia?" The idea had never crossed our minds, but we took the leap. On October 1, 2011, Keegan, Bradlee, my late mum, and I arrived in Australia. Karen and her husband, Oliver, joined us in January 2012.

When I arrived in Australia, I worked for an agency and my role was Manager of Children and Women's Services. My second job in Australia allowed me to work at a Women's Agency, supporting and managing client and children's safety after escaping domestic violence relationships. My third job at a large not-for-profit agency, I am a Manager of case workers who provide day to day case management for children in Out-of-Home Care.

After spending eight years in the Foster Care Industry and gaining a deep understanding of the needs of children, their foster carers, and the child protection system, I felt it would be beneficial to broaden my knowledge by learning about the NDIS System. My goal was to share this knowledge with my team, as well as with the children, birth parents, and foster carers. I had some basic knowledge as I began my research. I was curious about the policies and procedures of the NDIS. At one stage, I wanted to apply for a role in a government organisation. However, I could not continue my job application because I am a permanent resident of Australia and not a citizen. Employees at the NDIS are all citizens of Australia. I was curious about the Support Coordinator Role. The Support Coordinator Role is funded by the NDIS, and each client is allocated funding in their NDIS package to have a dedicated

Support Coordinator to assist with finding suitable support for the participant.

Exploring my son's NDIS Plan, I realised that the funding for his Support Coordinator had been allocated a while ago. However, I wondered about the Support Coordinator role – what exactly do they do? As a parent, I've diligently followed up on Keegan's medical reports, provided the NDIS with updated information, and obtained service quotes for the upcoming financial year to ensure the best possible funding approval to meet his needs.

Questions started piling up. Does the Support Coordinator only attend the annual NDIS Plan Review? With a busy full-time job, I kept putting off researching the details until I could find dedicated time to tackle the vast amount of information about how the NDIS System works for participants, parents, plan managers, support coordinators, funding types, what the NDIS funds, what it doesn't fund, and eligibility criteria.

Seeking answers, I attended a carers meeting where my son goes on weekdays. I raised concerns and questions about the Support Coordinator funding during the session. I inquired about how the budget is itemised, mainly since I handle most of the work for my son. Instead of receiving itemised billing, I get a service agreement with the total amount. Unfortunately, I have yet to receive a response at the time of writing this.

Having delved into questions about the Support Coordinator role and thoroughly researched the topic, I felt equipped with enough information to share with my team. My goal was to assist them in achieving the best outcomes for children in foster care through the NDIS. An essential realisation in this process is that NDIS employees decide how much and who is entitled to support coordination funding.

In my firm belief, if the budget is available for a child to have a support coordinator, parents, children, young people, and case managers must make enquiries for the child to receive the full range of funding from the NDIS. This ensures that children get the best support they need to thrive, relieving parents from the pressure of making countless phone calls to find therapists and specialists for their children. Despite being a practising Social Worker and a parent with a disabled son, I don't believe it's in my son's best interest to personally find support for him. Instead, I let his Support Coordinator handle this task since he has allocated funding. In consultation with him, I oversee the service agreements and determine the best way forward.

My focus and the best way forward seemed to be exploring how I could become an NDIS Provider to support families, their children, foster carers, and birth parents in navigating the NDIS effectively. I discovered different ways to subcontract from the NDIS, specifically as an unregistered or registered support coordinator.

To become a registered support coordinator, I realised I needed disability experience and qualifications that met the criteria for the specific services I wanted to provide to participants. I dedicated my after-work hours to reading up on NDIS material available on their website. Engaging in this research, learning new practice methods, and seeing all the puzzle pieces fit together was genuinely stimulating, and it gave me a deeper understanding of the NDIS.

After several months of thorough research and gathering information to support my NDIS Registered Provider application, I thought I had completed the task. However, finalising the paperwork proved to be an exciting journey. To become an NDIS Registered Provider, you must provide evidence for your application, including your Australian Business Number (ABN), copies of your degree, work history, driver's license, and trade name. Gathering all this paperwork took a few months.

The next step was to write up policies and procedures for my business. As I began this task, it became clear that it would take me much longer than expected. To streamline the process, I enlisted the help of an external company. Their expertise in policy writing and understanding of the NDIS proved invaluable in supporting me in reaching my goal. After reviewing five hundred pages of policies and procedures, I felt satisfied that the material aligned with the NDIS practice guidelines.

The next crucial step in the NDIS Business Registration process involves engaging an independent auditor. The auditor is tasked with conducting an external audit, providing recommendations to the prospective business owner seeking NDIS Provider Registration, and submitting the final decision on whether the Provider Registration will be approved by the NDIS. This audit process ensures that the business complies with the standards and practices outlined by the NDIS, contributing to the overall quality and reliability of services provided to NDIS participants.

In May 2023, I completed my NDIS Provider Registration and submitted it to the external auditor. In early July 2023, I met with the auditor to discuss my application, covering my work history, reasons for becoming a Specialist Support Coordinator with the NDIS, and how I aimed to help participants and their families find the best support for children to thrive. The audit was conducted offline, and although I was available for questions over the two days, I couldn't shake off the nervousness.

I received the news at the end of the second day – I passed the audit! The auditor had only made two minor recommendations, which I promptly addressed with no issues. My NDIS Provider Registration then proceeded to the NDIS for further scrutiny and the final outcome. I waited patiently, and three months later, I received an email from the NDIS confirming the success of my business application to become a registered NDIS Provider. This achievement marked another milestone in my life. I realised I could reach great heights personally and professionally through caring for my child, and his disability steered my curiosity to this point.

As an NDIS Registered Provider, I aim to maximise the benefits of the National Disability Insurance Scheme (NDIS) for children and clients, offering them the support and resources necessary to thrive. We recognise the significance of a comprehensive and personalised approach when navigating the complexities of the NDIS.

Allow us to assist you in getting the best out of the NDIS and ensuring that you or your loved ones receive the tailored support needed for a fulfilling life.

Facebook: – Kathleen Browne

Instagram: – Kathleen Browne

Personal and Professional Coaching for Parents – Join the most outstanding course – Mastering Special Needs Parenting – We Make It Work.

Closed Group on Facebook: The Unique Parent Club

CHAPTER 10

Balancing Work And Parenting

Even before I had children, I knew being a stay-at-home mum wasn't my path. I never envisioned myself staying at home, raising my kids, and finding fulfilment in parenthood. For me, fulfilment comes from having a career and being a parent simultaneously. The combination of professional growth and the joy of parenthood truly satisfies me.

As the parent of a child with special needs, my journey has been a constant emotional roller coaster as I strive to strike that delicate balance between my professional commitments and caregiving responsibilities. Through the highs and lows, I've understood the intricate emotional landscape I navigate daily. These emotions are not just mine; they are the shared experiences of countless parents in similar situations.

Facing challenges, I've always believed I'm not alone. Knowing others share similar struggles is an immense comfort. It's like having a community of parents who get our unique journey. Deep down, I find peace knowing family and friends are there to help if I need them. This support is a lifeline, a reassuring strength. Even in challenging moments, there are shoulders to lean on and hands to hold.

In those moments, it's easy to forget that help is available. You keep going, thinking you can catch up on sleep, time, and grocery shopping later. Sleep deprivation hit me hard when Keegan was born. The three-hour feeding schedule and constant monitoring took a toll. I put the paper away and told myself, "That's it. I can't keep doing this if I don't remember." I needed to do things my way, prioritise sleep, and feel better. Soon, I realised that I needed to sleep when Keegan slept too. Eventually, I settled into a sleeping routine with Keegan and learned the value of sleep. Until Bradlee came along. Bradlee was a good baby and sleeper; all he needed was to be fed, changed and sleep away.

Sleeping until the wee hours wasn't an option for me. Early rising and late nights were the norm for many years as I juggled work and parenting the boys. It takes time for kids to grow up. Then, one day, they no longer need you during the night or early morning. They cherish their sleep, maybe too much, especially during those teenage years.

Juggling drop-offs and school pickups was challenging, especially when the bus wasn't on time—stress levels hit the max. I planned my day carefully, allowing for some flexibility in case of delays. But sometimes I'd finish work and rush to the bus stop, and the bus was nowhere in sight. This happened in two countries I lived in: South Africa and New Zealand.

Having only one motorway in New Zealand meant any accident could leave you stranded. Fast travel became wishful thinking. You'd find yourself reading a book, chatting with a friend on the bus, or sneaking in a few winks to make the journey seem quicker. As I pondered what to do during these delays, I often pulled out my phone to set the 'late plan' in motion. Yes, you've got to have a late plan and call in the troops for help. It wasn't very often, but sometimes I needed to make that call.

I remember the day I had to make that call. I rang my sister, Karen, and asked her to pick up Keegan and Bradlee from after-school care. Karen, confused, wanted to know where I was. I explained I was stuck on a broken train, and it felt like it might be on fire. We weren't moving, and I did not know when I could pick up the boys from her place.

My story seemed unbelievable. In New Zealand, I always thought I'd take the express train, but that night, the express train was going nowhere. It was pouring rain, as it often does, and there we were, stuck on the train, waiting for updates on how we'd get home.

Finally, we were told to get off the train, climb down the side in the rain, and walk across the train lines to the platform. Then, we had to cross and join the next platform, where a train would pick us up to take us home. By then, it was dark, wet, and cold. Everyone followed the orders without complaint because our main goal was to get home as soon as possible. It took me two hours to get home that night. What a story it turned out to be! Nobody believed me when I told them the train broke down and was practically on fire with us on it.

In my wisdom, the next day, I drove to work, thinking I could avoid the hassles of public transport. I called my friend Kassy, and we planned to meet and travel home together in the afternoon. Little did I anticipate the woes that awaited us.

To my dismay, there was a traffic jam on the motorway heading to South Auckland, and diverting from the highway seemed futile as all roads were blocked. Going off the route wouldn't save us time, as we had no clue about the situation ahead. There were no radio reports, and we were stuck in a stationary vehicle on the motorway, waiting to go home.

That evening, I arranged for a taxi to pick up the boys from the after-school program. We all got home around the same time or in time. The plan was if I was later than the taxi, Bradlee would have a house key. He would open the door, lock it behind him, and wait for me to come home. Fortunately, this scenario didn't occur frequently. Most of the time, they made themselves a snack, watched television, and waited until I arrived.

Arriving late at work brought on a lot of stress, especially on mornings when I couldn't avoid it due to the kids oversleeping, tantrums, or Keegan having a rough night, sometimes even soiling himself and his bed. There was no stopping, and it felt like a constant juggling act.

I learned that when one of the boys threw a morning tantrum, I'd say, "Get your bags, shoes, and lunches. Let's go to the car.

I'm leaving and I will give you a honk when I leave. Please pull the door behind you so it locks, and we can head to the before-school program."

One morning, I started the car, honked, and opened the gate without response. Where were these boys? They had decided to sit and watch television and not budge an inch. Unfortunately, I couldn't leave them home alone, and there was no reason for me to stay home. So, I resorted to bribing them with their favourite meal for dinner—McDonald's. Off we all went to work and school in good spirits. I kept my word before you wonder what they had for dinner. I made buying dinner at McDonald's easier, giving myself a night off from kitchen duty.

When duty called, sometimes the nanny, who was supposed to be on duty, was late or didn't show up. I even had a nanny who got drunk on the job—yes, you read that right. In South Africa, nannies lived in the house, had a granny flat outside, or commuted from their homes daily.

One factor to consider was the time it took for the nanny to get to our home and the time she needed to leave in the afternoon to return to her place. When she exceeded her time, I'd start the car, put the boys in, and drive to the local train station. Her mode of transport often made her late, and on rare occasions, she didn't show up at all. She always had a seemingly reasonable excuse for her absence.

However, if I arrived home late, I would drive the nanny to the bus or train station, or sometimes even to her home, ensuring she could get there reasonably and spend time with her family. It was a delicate balance, considering both our responsibilities.

On this day, the nanny lived in the granny flat in our yard. Her family was in a different city, and she had friends in the area who were also nannies. I got a call from Bradlee's daycare, informing me that the school bus was at my home, but the nanny wasn't answering the doorbell, and there was no movement in the yard or house. I tried calling her repeatedly, but there was no answer. After several attempts, I informed my manager that I needed to take leave and find out what was happening with the nanny.

I arranged for Bradlee to be taken back to the daycare, and I would pick him up from there. Driving home with Bradlee, I realised I hadn't picked up Keegan. So, we went to get Keegan. To our surprise, when we got home and opened the house, there was no sign of the nanny. She wasn't anywhere in sight. I checked her granny's flat, used the spare keys to open the door, and found her passed out on the bed.

I called her name, and as I got closer, I could smell the alcohol. I tried to wake her, and she did, claiming she felt sick. I told her she needed to eat something and made it clear that I knew she was drunk, which was not okay with me. She had broken our trust.

Later, I discovered she had been drinking from the alcohol bottles in the bar and filling them up with water and black tea. I wouldn't have known if she hadn't decided to drink more than she could handle. The search for a new nanny began again.

Searching for a nanny was the last thing on my mind when we moved to New Zealand. My friend Kassy and I started taking the same bus to and from work. We became familiar faces on the bus, getting to know the drivers and fellow regulars. With so many acquaintances on the bus, I'd find someone else to chat with if she wasn't there.

I was surprised to find a long line at the bus stop one morning. Worried I had missed the bus, I was relieved to see Kassy waving from inside. She had saved me a seat so I didn't have to stand on the crowded bus to the city.

However, there was a twist. A man in front of me, who had boarded before I did, clipped his bus ticket and hurried to sit next to Kassy. As I walked down the aisle, I saw him in my spot. I smiled, hoping he would move, but he didn't. Instead, he declared, "You talk too much, and you don't need to talk to each other every day."

Kassy and I exchanged looks and started giggling, which seemed to annoy him even more because, try as he might, he couldn't stop us from chatting away. There was just too much to talk about, and he couldn't keep us quiet.

Balancing parenting and my career was challenging. I believe I did well. I can now relive and share those stories with my boys and readers. To all parents, I want to say that it gets easier.

There were moments of stress, like the worry of missing the bus when my friend was already on it. However, navigating through those challenges has provided me with stories to tell and lessons to share.

CHAPTER 11

Celebrating Milestones And Success

Celebrating a child's milestones has always been our tradition. Whether it's birthdays, the first tooth, the first haircut, the first steps, or the first day at daycare or school, these moments became a way of life for us. This tradition continued and became even more special with Keegan's busy schedule involving sports and school events.

In our everyday lives, we reach many milestones and find success. Yet, the small achievements of a child with special needs are significant accomplishments. We celebrate these moments with joy and laughter, making sure to treasure the memories. This is because, at the time of Keegan's birth, we had many questions about what he could do and what he might not achieve. I often wondered if he would walk, talk, make friends, and lead a fulfilling life. Today, it seems like he has, and he appears to be happy, savouring every moment of his life.

****

Keegan learned to walk.

Keegan learned to talk.

Keegan can feed himself.

Keegan can identify what he wants and what he does not want to do.

Keegan is aware of his surroundings.

Keegan loves his family, and they love him back.

Keegan has a favourite brother – only one, Bradlee.

Keegan has favourite Aunties; every day, they are numbered from one to four, and remember, Aunty number 4 is the Law. He knows.

Keegan has learned to choose his own clothes.

Keegan continues to learn how to shower and dry himself.

Keegan can put his shoes on the right way and sometimes he puts his sneakers on the wrong feet.

Keegan can brush his teeth and doesn't think it is necessary to comb his hair.

Keegan can help carry the groceries when he is in a good mood.

Keegan can push the shopping cart at the grocery store.

Keegan can eat with a knife and fork.

Keegan loves sitting on the floor. It is his place of comfort and relaxation.

Keegan loves his bed and his room and can spend time in his room doing whatever he loves to do now.

Keegan does not like going to bed, no matter how tired he is. I believe he thinks he will miss out on something. Every evening, we have the same routine and questions from him until he agrees to go to bed.

Keegan makes sure he sits in the front seat of the car. It is his spot. He appears to be grumpy when asked to sit at the back.

Keegan recognises every fast-food outlet we pass on the road. He loves McDonalds.

Keegan asks to visit his aunty's home because he knows where they keep the special treats.

Keegan does not swear, but when he has in the past, it makes me laugh, even though I shouldn't laugh. He hasn't said a bad word in years, or as long as I can remember.

Keegan knows his dad and his granny are in heaven.

Keegan loves checking out photos of himself on my phone, and he asked if he could have his own. I got a phone for him and am now busy adding pictures so he can have his collection on his phone.

Keegan is familiar with and can recognise the letters of the alphabet in his name. He can write his name when provided with a stencil, allowing him to trace over the lines.

Keegan can recognise places, houses, and landmarks and points these out as we drive through our neighbouring neighbourhoods.

Keegan can identify colours, and if we are travelling in the car and he is in a grumpy mood, we will spot the colours of the vehicles.

Keegan is the best travel companion in a car, train, bus, or aeroplane. While he has experienced sailing, we haven't been on a cruise ship together, and that's something we look forward to as it's on our bucket list.

Keegan loves music; he remembers the words of songs and would choose to sing instead of talk to me while I drive. Which is cool with me.

****

Reflecting on Keegan's milestones and achievements takes me back in time, remembering when he surprised me and my late husband by accomplishing new things. Holding his baby bottle was a milestone that took a bit longer for Keegan to achieve; he only started doing it when he was over a year old, realising he needed to hold it to be fed.

Celebrating Milestones And Success

Crawling came later for Keegan, well beyond his first year, mainly because he couldn't lie on his tummy due to his colostomy bag. His colostomy bag was removed when he was nine months old, marking a significant change. Afterwards, he had to learn to lie on his tummy, roll over, and take the following steps to reach his developmental milestones.

As Keegan learned to roll over, his legs and arms strengthened, and he became determined to move around. It was a slow process when he started crawling, and he favoured one side. I believe this might be linked to his tummy surgery, possibly still healing or causing discomfort. Despite this, he was determined to crawl and manoeuvre around the coffee table and the lounge suite. There were moments when it seemed he might give up, but he never did. His persistence and resilience were truly remarkable.

After many months of Keegan crawling and standing up, his dad bought him a wooden trolley and placed bricks in it for Keegan to push, strengthening his arm and leg muscles. Keegan enjoyed being outdoors and learned to push his trolley up and down the yard, gaining confidence and building his walking skills. It took nearly six months before he let go of the trolley handle and attempted to walk independently. We weren't in a rush; as long as he made an effort, it was a significant achievement to witness him giving his best.

One day, without any camera moment, I came home from work to find Keegan walking on his own. He did it when he was ready, without his trolleys or anyone else's support. He tried and succeeded, surprising us all with his determination and progress.

Keegan appeared in many school concerts.

He participated in school and Special Olympics athletics and shotput.

He enjoyed doing arts and crafts and came home with many drawings and coloured pages.

Keegan's most significant milestone was going on school camps. He loved being outdoors with his favourite school friends and teachers and took part as best he could.

Keegan and I learned to adjust to him staying away from home when he went into Respite Care. He always loved coming home and understands he can go to Respite Care when he spends time away from home and his mum.

Keegan attends his daily community program, where he participates in bowling, cooking, sailing, swimming, going to the pub for lunch and many more activities he enjoys.

Keegan is also willing to find work; his support team will help him achieve this huge milestone. If it is not soon, it will be in the future.

7 TIPS TO PLAN AND RECORD MEMORABLE MILESTONES FOR YOUR CHILD

PERSONAL CEREMONIES. You can organise small celebrations to highlight their achievements. Invite close family and friends and make a fuss while doing so, creating a moment in time and showcasing your child's journey.

MEMORY BOOKS OR PHOTO ALBUMS. These are valuable for you and for your child in the future. When Keegan takes out his albums, he recognises family members, his dad, his cousins in South Africa, friends in New Zealand, and extended family in Australia. It is a great way to capture their memories and remind them of their achievements.

ACTIVITIES AND SPECIAL OUTINGS. You can plan a special outing or activity that interests your child. These experiences create moments they will remember for a long time, especially if they highlight their unique abilities.

FOCUS ON YOUR CHILD'S STRENGTHS. Focussing on Keegan's strengths gives me power. I focus on what he can do in a day or month, his journey, and his journey for the past year. His learnings or development in the last year may be minimal. Yet, trying to do something different and improve is still his strength. Celebrating and complimenting him boosts his self-esteem and confidence.

FINDING JOY EVERY DAY. Sometimes, it is hard to find joy every day when you care and love your special needs child, especially when they are sick or just not doing their best that day. I usually try to think of a plan to get through the day, try to focus on what the result might be, and start working my way back to what is really happening in the moment so that I find joy at the end of any event, even if it was not as pleasant as Keegan or I hoped it to be.

CULTIVATE A POSITIVE MINDSET AND CELEBRATE RESILIENCE. I always try to think positively and see the positive or the learning experience from my parenting. Doing this gives me strength and motivates me to do better. Keegan is funny; he doesn't like to say the word 'no' and will answer everything I ask with a 'yes'. Did you brush your teeth? Keegan, did you shower, knowing full well that he didn't. Instead of fussing, I put toothpaste on his toothbrush, opened the shower taps, watched the water temperature gauge, and walked away. Once, I heard the water running and didn't hear any splashing or asking me for soap, only to go back into Keegan's bathroom; he was leaning over the bathroom sink and looking at himself in the mirror. I had to ask him to get on with his personal care, and he responded, "No, you do it." Cheeky.

NURTURING SIBLING RELATIONSHIPS. It was challenging for me to nurture Keegan and Bradlee's relationships. There is a five-year age gap between them, and they are different. They had their own personalities, likes, dislikes, and loved each other endlessly when they were little, and they still have a great bond and love for each other. The challenge, I suppose, is when the sibling without the disability makes friends outside of the family circle, goes out and does teenage stuff with their friends, it can sometimes be difficult for siblings to remain in the same friendship circle. However, I did not need to nurture the boy's relationship regarding Bradlee attending events for Keegan. He was at the rugby games, school concerts, special Olympic events, and dances, dropping off and picking up Keegan from events with me and making friends with Keegan's friends. I think it is more accessible for sibling relationships to work if both siblings are doing stuff together. It does not mean they need to be together all the time just because one of the siblings has a disability. I find that with my two boys, there is always the protective factor for Keegan. Bradlee is constantly checking on him and ensuring he is ok. Keegan waits for Bradlee's reaction and is always happy to see him.

Fostering positive sibling relationships provides a supportive and understanding family dynamic. Let us continue to celebrate and embrace special needs children, appreciating their unique abilities and contributions to our lives.

CHAPTER 12

Future Planning

Growing up, the importance of future planning was instilled in me. Even as an eighteen-year-old, my late mother emphasised the necessity of taking out a Funeral Policy. It may sound sombre, but the truth is, without a solid plan for the future, my life and the lives of my children would have been thrown into disarray when their father passed away suddenly. Discussing or writing about such matters is never easy. Still, I believe sharing my thoughts and experiences with you is crucial. Future planning, particularly for Keegan and Bradlee, always remains a top priority. It not only simplifies my life and reduces stress but also provides assurance that they will be cared for when I am no longer around. This is especially vital for Keegan, who requires an additional plan to support him throughout the rest of his life.

FINANCIAL PLANNING FOR THE FUTURE

When I was younger, saving was difficult because I wanted to buy beautiful clothes, shoes, handbags and earrings. It was just what I and other young girls did in my day. However, life changes when you have children. Your financial decisions change because prioritising expenditure is one challenge we all need to overcome by learning to respect the incoming finances, be grateful for the amounts received and then channel the quantities to the correct accounts or beneficiaries to reduce everyday stress, worries, sleepless nights, and know there is a little tucked away for a rainy day.

Rainy days come along, and I experienced a fair share of those, especially when my family and I moved to different countries, changed jobs, or needed to stay home and care for my boys on a single income. Life teaches us different ways to prioritise what we do at the moment. It was eye-opening for me when I went from being part of a two income family to a one income family. I needed to learn and to ensure I provided for my boys so they could live the same lifestyle their father and I chose for them.

It was not a lavish lifestyle. It was, however, a lifestyle to be educated, learn respect for others, challenge the status quo if needed, and always ensure you believed in someone or something higher than yourself. By this, I mean having faith in God, that he will provide, and belief in yourself to make it happen. I needed to rely on my faith often to know that my financial gains or ills were my doing. I learnt ways to correct them quickly. In that learning, I began understanding the importance of financial planning for the future.

Financial planning is a crucial link to life management. From an early age, I learned the importance of looking ahead, ensuring I had measures to navigate life's uncertainties; however, sometimes, I was caught off guard when I strayed from the plan. While it might seem daunting to talk about or consider life insurance or retirement savings, addressing these topics, head-on is taking a proactive approach to safeguarding your future and that of your child with special needs.

Reflecting on my journey, I can attest to the peace of mind of having a comprehensive financial plan. It goes beyond mere budgeting; it involves thoughtful consideration of investments, emergency funds, and retirement strategies. The foresight to plan for unexpected events, such as illness or unforeseen expenses, has proven invaluable.

Sharing this perspective is not meant to dwell on morbid subjects, but to underscore the relevance of financial planning in our lives. By making informed decisions and setting financial goals, I secure my future and ensure that my loved ones, like Keegan and Bradlee, have a safety net. It's a proactive approach that not only eases the current stresses but also lays the foundation for a more secure future.

LEGAL GUARDIANSHIP OPTIONS

I recently visited my lawyer to update my living will and complete an Enduring Power of Attorney and a Guardianship Order. Completing these forms and documents takes time and energy, and careful planning of what I want for myself should anything happen to me. While I am clear about who will carry out my wishes at the end of my life, I always worry about who will care for Keegan when I am no longer around.

I don't think I am the only parent with a special needs adult son who feels this way. We all think this way, and I will assume that all parents think this way even if you don't think of it now or when you just have kids. The question will come up at some stage. You will ask yourself, *Who will care for my kids when I am gone?* It is not a simple question to answer because you don't have a crystal ball to see into the future on how your life and your children's lives will play out and who will take care of them. You need to know that there are good people in the world who will take care of your children. These could be family, friends, neighbours, or community members who can and will do it because we all need care, love and attention irrespective of how old and long we live.

When we lived in New Zealand, it was vital for me to apply for Legal Guardianship for Keegan, as there was a need for the New Zealand Government to ensure Keegan's rights and responsibilities were taken into account when decisions were made for him. At first, I was distraught because I felt my parenting had been undermined, and Keegan needed a piece of paper from the court that said he could live with me and I could make decisions for him. Imagine that!

Although the initial thought surprised me, the shock started wearing off. I was in a better place to receive the information and understand why the New Zealand Government requested me to complete this critical step for Keegan, as it would not only be part of his life. We would all become citizens of New Zealand as a family.

During the process of applying for legal guardianship for Keegan, he met with a lawyer, I met with the lawyer, and the lawyer needed to speak with his school, family members and the wider community who knew Keegan and me to ensure there was an established relationship between Keegan and me. It was a long wait, and after the matter was listed for hearing, the court granted me guardianship for Keegan. I was not really stressed or phased about the process because deep down in my heart, I knew there was no way the court could deny me the right to care for my child. That's me and the strength I needed to endure this process.

However, the process in Australia is very different. When I asked my lawyer if I needed to apply for a guardianship order for Keegan, his words were, "Why?". I explained to him the position I was in when we lived in New Zealand, and he let me know in Australia, you can apply for a Guardianship Order to care for your adult child. However, the social service agencies we are in contact with have never asked me to show or prove I have legal guardianship for Keegan.

In Australia, I need to constantly complete nomination forms, where Keegan makes me a nominee on his Centrelink, Workforce Australia, National Disability Insurance Scheme (NDIS) and many more companies and agencies who need assurance that he has a parent or carer to take care of him and make decisions for him.

However, I sometimes find this process frustrating as so much paperwork is never-ending. At times, with some agencies, there is a constant reminder that information needs to be updated. Each year, I need to complete nomination forms for Keegan. I sometimes wonder if it would be easier to go to the court and apply for Guardianship and give them the documents to prove that I, Keegan's parent, can care for him and act on his behalf. I am still not sure about this, and perhaps one day, the systems for people with a disability will collide and I will only complete one form for all agencies.

A legal representative or your lawyer can explain the implications of legal guardianship, as it was in my case with Keegan. Knowing what the guardianship order involves and finding guardians to care for your child is a parent's choice and your child's choice if they can understand and voice their views on what they believe is in their best interest.

FAMILY SUPPORT NETWORK

As I discussed how crucial it is to have a family support network, I emphasise this to ensure the well-being of your son or daughter in the event of your demise. Keegan and Bradlee's dad died suddenly when they were eight and three years old. Without my family's support, I would not have been able to cope with our challenges. Keegan's disability made it harder for him to understand mortality. Although Bradlee was three years old, he knew his dad was not coming back and only grasped what mortality really meant at a later stage in his life.

I know, and I have this gut feeling in me that if something happens to me, Keegan will go and live with his brother, Bradlee, or live with one of my sisters, or he has an option of updating his NDIS plan and having sufficient funding to go and live in Supported Disability Accommodation (SDA). I am happy Keegan has options, and even though I will not be around to see how all this plays out for Keegan should I pass on before him, I know that he will be cared for because there are people in my family, his dad's family, his brother, and his aunties and his uncle in Australia will take him in and care for him the same way I do. I know this for sure and am strengthened by these thoughts.

By establishing a solid support network for yourself and your child, you can ensure your child's needs are met even when you can no longer provide for them. Keeping and strengthening family bonds and creating a network for yourself and your child is vital.

COMMUNITY RESOURCES AND SERVICES

When you are no longer around to provide assistance and support to your disabled son, it is crucial to identify community resources and services that can step in and offer the help he needs. These resources can be vital in ensuring your son receives the care and support he requires.

Several programs, organisations, and government initiatives offer specialised care for disabled individuals. These resources cater to the unique needs of individuals like your son, providing them with the necessary support to lead fulfilling lives.

One such resource is disability-specific support organisations. These organisations are dedicated to advocating for individuals with disabilities and providing services such as counselling, support groups, educational programs, and social activities. They can offer your son a supportive community and access to resources to enhance his quality of life.

Government initiatives also play a significant role in assisting individuals with disabilities. Depending on your location, government-funded programs may offer financial aid, healthcare services, and vocational training for disabled individuals. These programs aim to empower individuals with disabilities and enable them to live independently and participate fully in society.

Exploring local community resources such as community centres, recreational facilities, and non-profit organisations is essential. These resources often offer various programs and services tailored to the needs of individuals with disabilities, including sports activities, art classes, and therapy services. Engaging in such activities can promote socialisation, skill development, and overall well-being for your son.

Remember to seek out and make connections with other families who have children with disabilities. Support groups and online communities can be valuable sources of information and emotional support. These families can provide insights into local resources and share their experiences navigating the various services available for disabled individuals.

CREATING A CARE PLAN

Creating a comprehensive care plan for your disabled son is crucial for ensuring that his specific needs, preferences, and routines are met even when you can no longer provide direct care. Following a step-by-step approach, you can develop a care plan addressing all aspects of your son's well-being.

First, assess your son's needs, considering his physical, cognitive, emotional, and social requirements. Consult with healthcare professionals, therapists, and educators who have worked closely with your son to gain a comprehensive understanding of his abilities and limitations.

Next, outline the specific services and support your son requires. This may include medical care, therapy sessions, educational support, personal care assistance, and social activities. Consider these services' frequency, duration, and intensity to ensure they align with your son's needs.

It is essential to involve your son in the care planning process to the extent possible. Consider his preferences, interests, and routines. This will help maintain a sense of autonomy and promote his overall well-being. Regularly review and update the care plan as your son's needs and circumstances evolve.

Collaboration and coordination with healthcare professionals, therapists, educators, and others involved in your son's care are crucial. Establish open lines of communication to ensure that everyone is aware of the care plan and can work together effectively to meet your son's needs.

Lastly, consider the financial and legal aspects of the care plan. Explore financial resources, such as disability benefits and insurance coverage, to help cover services and support costs. Consult with an attorney specialising in disability law to ensure appropriate legal measures are in place to protect your son's rights and ensure his care plan is upheld.

Regularly reviewing and updating the care plan is essential to ensure its effectiveness. As your son grows and experiences changes in his abilities and circumstances, adjustments may be necessary to meet his evolving needs. By staying proactive and engaged in the care planning process, you can provide your disabled son with the best possible care and support throughout his life.

FINANCIAL PLANNING FOR LONG-TERM CARE: SECURING A STABLE FUTURE FOR YOUR DISABLED CHILD

Planning for the long-term care of a disabled child after your passing is an essential aspect of financial planning.

Financial Considerations for Long-Term Care

SPECIAL NEEDS TRUST

A special needs trust is a powerful tool that allows you to set aside funds for your disabled child's long-term care while preserving their eligibility for government benefits. By establishing a special needs trust, you can ensure their financial needs are met even after your passing.

GOVERNMENT BENEFITS

Understanding and maximising government benefits is crucial for securing financial stability in the long run. Programs like Supplemental Security Income (SSI) and Medicaid provide financial assistance and healthcare coverage for disabled individuals. Researching and applying for these benefits can significantly ease the financial burden of long-term care.

LIFE INSURANCE POLICIES

Life insurance can provide a safety net for your child's financial future. By choosing a policy with suitable coverage, you can ensure sufficient funds are available to cover their long-term care needs. It is essential to consult with a financial advisor to determine the appropriate coverage amount and type of policy.

ESTATE PLANNING

Proper estate planning ensures that your assets are distributed according to your wishes. Creating a comprehensive estate plan lets you specify how your child's long-term care expenses will be covered. This may include designating funds for their care, appointing a guardian or trustee, and outlining instructions for managing their finances.

STRATEGIES FOR SECURING FINANCIAL STABILITY

SEEK PROFESSIONAL ADVICE

Consulting with financial advisors, estate planners, and special needs attorneys can provide valuable guidance on navigating long-term care's complex financial planning landscape. These professionals can help you understand the options, evaluate your financial situation, and develop a customised plan that meets your child's needs.

REGULARLY REVIEW AND UPDATE FINANCIAL PLANS

Financial circumstances and government regulations may change over time. It is essential to regularly review and update your financial plans to ensure they remain aligned with your goals. This includes assessing the adequacy of your savings, evaluating investment strategies, and staying informed about any changes to government benefits that may affect your child's financial situation.

CHAPTER 13

Life Lessons Learned

Wisdom Gained Through Experience and Reflection

Reflecting on the challenges I faced in giving birth to a child with a disability, I can now appreciate that I gave my best with the resources and time available to me. Navigating the uncharted territory of parenting a child with special needs presented me with a series of unknowns. Still, I confronted these uncertainties with resilience and determination.

As I realised that there was no turning back for myself and my child, it became clear that embracing the journey was essential. I needed to turn my unique path of special needs parenting into something that worked specifically for me. This revelation dawned upon me early in my baby's life, prompting the understanding that I had to make this extraordinary journey survivable and a source of personal growth.

This epiphany marked a crucial turning point. I recognised the importance of tailoring my approach to suit my needs, not conforming to external expectations. It was about crafting a path that worked for me and my child, acknowledging the uniqueness of our situation. In embracing this mindset early on, I laid the foundation for a journey that was not just about coping but about thriving in the face of the unknowns associated with special needs parenting.

RECOGNISE YOUR RESILIENCE

I was once asked by a close associate, "How do you do this all on your own, and you don't even have a husband?". Having a husband does not make me a good parent. Or deny me the privilege to do things on my own. Having been parented by two remarkable parents and shown, guided, and coached throughout my life makes me know I was loved and cared for. I belonged to a part of a wider group who knew me, knew what I was capable of, and knew I could do anything, even in the face of adversity.

I can assure you having a child with special needs taught me how to navigate through various obstacles and setbacks. It is not an easy road to travel. However, through the journey, I developed a remarkable level of resilience. I learned to bounce back from any unexpected circumstance, find the inner strength to face my challenges head-on and come out at the other end with new skills, knowledge and understanding until the next challenge comes along.

I recognise my resilience daily and learn how to manage situations from the past and daily. I remember my strength of working through my grief after the sudden loss of my husband, an immediate change in my financial situation and how I learnt to manage on a single income, having learned how to be a single parent, pack up and move and setting up home in two totally different countries, having to learn how to be true to myself. I know what is good and what is not suitable for me at this age. I learnt to say, "it is not ok for me," when asked to do something that does not align with my values and beliefs. I knew that my resilience came from within me, and only I could control myself. No person in this wide world can change my strength to love, care for, and be me except me.

Recognising your resilience is one way to keep you strong.

EMOTIONAL GROWTH

My emotional growth developed and matured as I learned different ways of doing things, understood the importance of parenting, and managed my emotions in different situations. When I think about my emotional growth, I think about nurturing a garden within me. A garden requires me to tend to it and cultivate it to produce a dynamic landscape. This takes patience, self-awareness, self-regulation, empathy, interpersonal skills, resilience, positive coping mechanisms, and emotional maturity. However, and I say however, dynamic growth paths are different to each person.

I can attest there are times in my life and even to this day that sometimes my emotions are tested, when I cannot recognise my resilience and when I may not have the patience to manage or deal with a particular situation because I feel hurt, betrayed or totally ignored even when I express how I feel.

Recognising my self-awareness and telling myself I did not do okay in that situation is complex. You need to make it right. You need to check if you are ok. What I mean is that there are times when I cannot say something is white when it is black, and I can sure as hell tell you it is black because I know it is black, and you cannot convince me otherwise. What I mean here is that I know for sure what is accurate, and in the event of us having a conversation, I am told that is invalid. I find it challenging to continue the conversation because it would mean I believe your lie, especially when I cannot be a party to deceit and wrongdoing. Perhaps I am scared of the law. Maybe I do not want to go to prison. Perhaps the times when I cannot regulate myself and not follow someone else's path are correct for me.

As I navigate life's challenges, and each experience makes me more robust, more self-aware and more resilient in my coping, I also develop my communication skills and empathy towards others in my family and the wider community. I have also developed emotional maturity, demonstrating balance and thoughtful approaches to emotional situations, considering that sometimes a parent of a special needs child's patience is tested by bureaucratic forms and long wait times for medical appointments.

Bringing a balance of thought and emotions to a situation makes life less stressful and enjoyable. It can also get me further in my emotional growth plan, so I do not take two steps forward and one step back. Emotional growth is not a linear process. It is a continuous journey of love, hate, friendship, stress, challenges, and planning. All the while, we learn more and more about ourselves to reach a higher point where we can say we did it.

I am also aware growing emotionally requires me to reflect, learn and adapt. This approach has always been at the heart of my personal and professional growth and development plan. In my personal life, I travelled abroad with trainers who have come before me to share their knowledge and skills and what they have overcome to build an empire and make a difference in the world. In my professional career, I too have learned, gone back to university to build my knowledge so that I know how to support people in my community and do the best I can with the information I learnt, all the while continuing the journey of learning to become emotionally in tune with the world and those around me.

APPRECIATION AND CULTIVATION OF SELF-ADVOCACY SKILLS

I have always been a good advocate for myself and believe that social justice is ingrained in my DNA, which I cannot deny. Giving birth to a child with special needs and raising him into an adult male has afforded me the appreciation of learning to cultivate my self-advocacy skills.

I reflect on my strengths and personal and professional values and determine which goals suit me while caring for my adult son. Self-reflection takes practice, dedication, and time to stop and think about what is happening in your life and what you have learnt on that day or moment. It allows me time to identify a specific situation where I have struggled, navigate the struggle and advocate for myself if I have not done so in the past.

I learned to educate myself on my rights in various contexts, such as education, employment and healthcare. While I advocate for Keegan's rights in the Disability arena, it is also essential for me to remind myself that I, too, need to think about myself and know the rights of the countries where I live. Navigating the education sector and understanding employment conditions and healthcare practices in three countries has been an enormous learning experience. Knowledge in these areas allows me to converse confidently with stakeholders in higher positions who make decisions for me and Keegan.

While it is important to educate myself in different areas of practice, I also learned to clarify my needs, define my goals and understand the information before making a request. I know that not all my proposals will be met in my favour. However, having the patience to understand why something was not approved at my request gives me hope for a different way to travel to fulfil my goal. To do this, I must prioritise what is most important, as I cannot simultaneously work on too many projects.

In appreciating and recognising my self-advocacy skills, I learned to build my confidence, set boundaries, seek information and resources, and solve problems when they arise. If there is one thing that I like to do for myself and others is to solve problems. I have always had this innate ability to solve problems, and I am unsure how I learned this skill. I believe I was born with it, and I worked with a colleague who said to me one day,

"How do you do that? How can you work out an issue so quickly and come up with a resolution?"

I said, "I don't know, I just do it and don't realise I am doing it."

She mentioned, "It is a good skill to have."

In saying that, over the years, I have honed in on my self-advocacy skills and learned to stay persistent in my parenting, advocating for my rights, understand setbacks as a natural part of the learning process, learn from the challenges, take them on head-on, and move to the next level in life where I feel more fulfilled, hopeful and have faith knowing I can do it.

In special needs parenting, advocating for your child becomes a necessity. Parents learn to navigate complex systems, communicate effectively with professionals, and stand up for their children's rights. This journey enables parents to develop invaluable self-advocacy skills that extend beyond their role as a parent.

PRACTISING SELF-CARE

I always knew how to take care of my physical and emotional health. However, as time passed, I learned about practising self-care and what it genuinely meant for it to become part of my life. I needed to recognise that while I was good at practising some areas of self-care in my life, I also needed to learn other areas that I did not concentrate on or was totally not interested in learning or practising.

Even when writing my book, I needed to stop and reflect on which areas I practice self-care and which I don't. I know for sure that:

I PRIORITISE MY SLEEP

Prioritising sleep is a crucial aspect of my daily routine, ensuring I maintain physical mobility and mental alertness to fulfil my responsibilities as a parent and work towards my goals. I adhere to a consistent sleep routine, striving to secure seven uninterrupted hours of sleep on most nights. Even when my bedtime is disrupted, I make a conscious effort to compensate by going to bed earlier the following night and maintaining a commitment to sufficient sleep.

While I value the importance of rest, I face the challenge of being unable to linger in bed once I wake up. This inclination, rooted in my preference for an early start, contrasts with the sleep-in habits preferred by my family, particularly during holidays. Despite their desire for a more leisurely morning, my internal clock prompts me to rise early. I recognise the potential for adjusting this aspect of my routine to accommodate differing preferences. However, doing so may lead to a delayed start to my day, potentially impacting my ability to accomplish essential tasks.

Navigating this balance between prioritising sleep and adapting to varying schedules remains a consideration. Perhaps finding a middle ground that allows for restful mornings without compromising productivity could be explored, offering a compromise that aligns with personal well-being and daily life's practical demands.

I CONNECT WITH OTHERS

I have a large family, and we keep in regular contact. I have Keegan's community, with whom I keep in touch. I like to stay in touch with people who uplift me and encourage me to fulfil my goals and do better for myself. My sisters and brothers are good supporters as they are always around to help me in my time of need and listen to me when I need to talk through a challenge to make the best decision for myself.

I ALWAYS SEEK SUPPORT

Seeking support is my priority, especially if I need to contact government and non-government departments to support me, find out information, and know the rules. It is asking for help. I try not to hesitate to ask for help from friends, family or support groups when needed. Sometimes, when I engage in learning or completing a course, I understand from others that the service I need may come from different sources, not only family, friends and people I know.

I STAY ORGANISED

I learned to be organised from a young age. I have six siblings, and our household was very organised. I did not grow up in a show home. Our home was our home, yet everything was in its place. We slept on double bunks, had a draw for our personal items, and shared a wardrobe. Having older siblings and a mum who taught me to be organised has helped me maintain my sanity; significantly raising a child with special needs, I needed to adapt the way I manage my life and the way my home is organised to accommodate my children and still find spaces for them to make them feel comfortable in their own home.

I SET REALISTIC GOALS

On reflection, I recognised I always set one goal that I believe at the time may not be realistic; however, when I work on the project or managing my time better, I can get down to meeting the targets I set for myself in completing the goal. One example I have is writing a book, which has always been on my to-do list; one day, I realised it was time to complete this goal because it was always something I wanted to do, and eventually, I did it. It is an outstanding achievement when you complete a mammoth task, such as becoming a published author.

Before I go on and share what I am not good at when practising self-care, I also note that I take short breaks and go away on weekends and longer holidays to recharge and return feeling better. I love gardening when I have the time, and it gives me great satisfaction when the plants grow and the garden is in bloom. When I bloom and achieve success, I celebrate my achievements because they give me the strength to complete the next milestone.

Thinking and writing about what I don't do well is ok with me because I know I am always working towards becoming more equipped in self-care.

I don't exercise regularly, practice mindfulness, or create a relaxing environment in my home. I am candid about this: I find it hard to exercise regularly, even to go for a 30-minute walk around the block. Yet when I was younger, I went to the gym and loved to dance and go for long walks in the area, and all this was put in the too-hard basket because I didn't set up a routine to do it. I simply ignore it and hope it is going to go away.

I always hear people say they practice mindfulness and meditation, which helps them reduce stress. I have tried meditation in the past and can still do it if I choose to do it; however, it is not part of my routine, and I find I would instead read to reduce stress, talk to someone on the phone or connect with another person. I love my company and being on my own when I get the time, which is hard when you have children. However, being alone recharges me because I can concentrate on something I want to do for those hours or minutes.

I try to create a calm and restful home environment, which is a work in progress; however, I don't have a designated space in my home that I believe is the best place to relax. I feel I can relax sitting at my computer, reading a book or cooking a meal. I may resist having a designated space to relax because I may not have the time to go and sit in that space or room to ponder my thoughts. I will undoubtedly work towards this self-care goal. Hopefully, one day, I will fully understand the beauty of this action.

Although there are different practices on how we care for ourselves, mentally and physically, there is more to self-care than I can write about today. Taking care of myself will allow me to be healthy and live a more balanced life. However, I don't think about it too much or stress because we are all different; indeed, no one size fits in the fantastic realm of life. What works for one person may certainly not work for me. It is about finding what works and what I hope to work towards in managing and balancing my self-care responsibilities.

Reflecting on personal growth and resilience gained through special needs parenting is essential to acknowledge the strength and determination it requires. By embracing the journey, finding joy amidst the challenges, and planning for the transition to adulthood, parents can nurture their own growth while supporting their child's development. Through resilience, advocacy, and unwavering love, parents can create a brighter future for their child with special needs.

About The Author

Enthusiastic Entrepreneur, Compassionate Mum, Full-Time Carer, Social Worker, Life Coach, and NDIS Registered Provider – a story of resilience, compassion, and the unwavering pursuit of making a difference.

In the vibrant tapestry of life, Kathleen Browne's journey as a business owner and life coach unfolds as a natural progression in pursuit of her life's purpose. Today, she proudly spearheads Kathleen Browne, Social Work Services and Tweelie, an NDIS-registered organisation, navigating the extraordinary path alongside parents of children with special needs.

Kathleen is not one to rest; instead, she seeks solutions and actively makes a difference for those who turn to her for support. Her unique perspective stems from personal experience — at the age of twenty-five, her first child was diagnosed with Down Syndrome. When her husband passed away at 34, Kathleen assumed the primary parenting role, setting her on a transformative course. She not only learned to support her son but also returned to university, becoming a Social Worker with an insider's view of the support systems for people with disabilities.

Having lived in three countries, Kathleen adeptly navigated bureaucracy, immigration intricacies, and disability legislation, constantly working towards enhancing the lives of children. Today, she shares her life story, detailing the challenges and triumphs of raising her son both with and without her beloved husband. Kathleen's narrative is candid, baring her soul to convey the often-difficult reality of being a single parent of a child with a disability.

With over two decades of professional experience, Kathleen's background includes managing corporate teams in the financial industry. As a program manager in an out-of-home care organisation, she supported foster carers and children with and without diagnosed disabilities in out-of-home care.

Kathleen's unwavering commitment to social justice is ingrained in her DNA. Her astute advocacy skills and self-determination qualities shine through, enriching her book and workshop development. Through her writing and workshops, Kathleen extends a guiding hand to parents navigating the extraordinary journey of raising children with special needs, making the seemingly challenging path appear effortlessly manageable.

Join The Unique Parent Club With Kathleen Browne

Embarking on the journey of parenting a special needs child can be both challenging and rewarding. Kathleen Browne, the author of 'The Unique Parent Club,' extends a warm invitation to parents navigating this unique path. Here's how you can get started on this transformative journey:

JOIN THE UNIQUE PARENT CLUB

Connect with a community of parents who understand the intricacies of raising special needs children. This club is not just run by parents; it's created for parents. Share experiences, gain insights, and build a supportive network.

SIGN UP WITH KATHLEEN BROWNE

Engage with an NDIS Registered Provider and benefit from the expertise of a Specialist Service Coordinator. Connect on Facebook and Instagram to stay informed, ask questions, and be part of a community that thrives on shared knowledge and experiences.

FREE PLANNED NDIS PLAN HEALTH CHECK

We understand the challenges of navigating the NDIS for your child. That's why we're excited to offer you a FREE Planned NDIS Plan Health Check! Ensure your child's plan aligns perfectly with their needs and unlocks the support they deserve. Ready to take the next step? Claim your FREE Health Check now! Your child's brighter future starts here.

BOOK A 15-MINUTE COACHING SESSION

Personalised guidance can make a significant difference. Book a coaching session with Kathleen to address specific concerns, seek advice, or clarify your unique parenting journey.

SUBSCRIBE AND JOIN MINI-SEMINARS

Stay informed and inspired by subscribing to Mini-Seminars. Explore a wealth of knowledge on parenting special needs children, delivered directly to you.

CONTACT KATHLEEN FOR SPEAKING ENGAGEMENTS

If you're organising an event and would like an expert perspective on Disability Parenting, the NDIS, and insights from the Unique Parent Club, reach out to Kathleen. Her experiences and wisdom can provide valuable insights to your audience.

BE UPDATED ON PARENTING RETREATS

Take a break, rejuvenate, and connect with other parents at Parenting Retreats. Stay updated on upcoming retreats for an opportunity to relax, learn, and share in a supportive environment.

SIGN UP - RAISING SPECIAL NEEDS CHILDREN – A PARENTING COACHING PROGRAM

Explore the comprehensive Parenting Coaching Program explicitly designed for raising special needs children. Gain practical tools, insights, and ongoing support to navigate the challenges and joys of your unique parenting journey.

Join the Unique Parent Club today and let Kathleen Browne be your guide and companion on this extraordinary parenting adventure.

The Unique Parent Club

Chapter 1: Introduction to the Unique Parent Club

The Unique Parent Club is an exclusive organisation that celebrates and supports the diversity of parenting experiences.

1.1 Background

Parenting is a universal experience that comes with its own set of challenges and joys. However, every parent's journey is unique, influenced by various factors such as culture, location, and personal circumstances. Recognising this, the Unique Parent Club was established to create a space where parents from all walks of life can come together, share their stories, and find support.

1.2 Mission Statement

The mission of the Unique Parent Club is to foster inclusivity, respect, and understanding among parents of diverse backgrounds. We aim to create a supportive community where all parents can connect, learn from each other, and celebrate the rich tapestry of special needs parenting experiences.

1.3 Objectives

To achieve our mission, the Unique Parent Club focuses on the following objectives:

1.3.1 Providing a Supportive Network: We strive to build a strong network of parents who can offer one another emotional support, guidance, and practical advice. Through online forums, local meetups, and virtual events, we create opportunities for parents to connect and form meaningful relationships.

1.3.2 Sharing Parenting Resources: We believe in the power of knowledge-sharing. The Unique Parent Club offers various resources, including articles, webinars, and workshops, covering different aspects of parenting. From newborn care to adolescent development, we aim to equip parents with valuable information to navigate their unique parenting journeys.

1.3.3 Promoting Cultural Exchange: The Unique Parent Club values diversity and cultural exchange. We encourage parents to share their cultural traditions, practices, and perspectives, fostering a deeper understanding and appreciation of different parenting approaches worldwide.

1.3.4 Advocating for Parental Rights: We recognise the importance of advocating for the rights and well-being of parents. The Unique Parent Club actively engages in discussions and initiatives to influence policies and practices that impact parents' lives.

1.4 Benefits of Joining

By becoming a member of the Unique Parent Club, parents gain access to a range of benefits, including:

- Exclusive access to a supportive community of parents from diverse backgrounds
- Opportunities to connect with other parents through local meetups and virtual events
- Access to a wealth of parenting resources, including articles, webinars, and workshops
- Discounts on relevant products and services
- The chance to contribute to discussions and initiatives that shape the future of parenting

1.5 Conclusion

In conclusion, the Unique Parent Club is a vibrant and inclusive community that celebrates the uniqueness of every parent. By joining our club, parents can find support, gain knowledge, and connect with others who share their parenting journey.

A Parenting Coaching Program

RAISING SPECIAL NEEDS CHILDREN

Empower your journey as a parent with our Mastering Special Needs Parenting Coaching Program. Join a community of support, gain expert insights, and discover the tools to navigate the extraordinary path of parenting a child with special needs. Sign up now and embark on a transformative adventure towards greater understanding, resilience, and joy. Your family's extraordinary story deserves exceptional guidance – let's master it together!

Introduction:

Welcome to a transformative coaching journey designed exclusively for parents navigating the unique challenges of raising children with special needs. This comprehensive package offers support, guidance, and a roadmap to help you shift from moments of *heartbreak to a life filled with joy, connection, and newfound strength.*

Package Overview:

1. Discovery Session: Unveiling Your Strengths and Resilience

In this foundational session, we'll explore your unique strengths as a parent and cultivate resilience to empower you on this journey. Together, we'll lay the groundwork for positive transformation.

2. Navigating the Emotional Landscape: Strategies for Coping and Thriving

Understand, manage, and transcend the emotional rollercoaster that often accompanies parenting a child with special needs. Learn practical strategies to foster emotional well-being for both you and your child.

3. Creating a Supportive Environment: Build Your Tribe

Cultivate a strong support network by connecting with other parents with similar experiences. Discover the power of community, share insights, and build lasting connections that will sustain and uplift you.

4. Advocacy Mastery: Championing Your Child's Needs

Equip yourself with practical advocacy skills to ensure your child receives the best educational, medical, and social support. Learn how to navigate systems, communicate effectively, and become a powerful advocate for your child.

5. Building Resilient Family Dynamics: Fostering Sibling Bonds

Strengthen family bonds and create an inclusive environment where every member feels valued. Explore activities and communication strategies to foster healthy relationships among siblings and family members.

6. Holistic Self-Care: Nurturing Your Well-being

Develop a personalised self-care plan prioritising your physical, emotional, and mental well-being. Recharge and rediscover joy in everyday moments, ensuring you have the energy and resilience to support your child.

7. Setting and Celebrating Milestones: Your Child's Unique Journey

Explore realistic goal-setting for your child and celebrate their achievements, no matter how small. Learn to appreciate the uniqueness of your child's journey and find joy in their progress.

8. Future Planning: Empowering Your Child for Independence

Strategies for the future by exploring options for your child's independence and well-being. Navigate transitions smoothly, whether transitioning to adulthood, independent living, or vocational pursuits.

Summing up:

Embark on this empowering coaching journey that promises to transform *heartbreak into happiness*. Together, we'll navigate the intricate tapestry of parenting exceptional children, *embracing the joys, overcoming challenges*, and building *a future filled with hope and fulfilment*.

The Unique Parent Club

Are you ready to transform your parenting experience and *cultivate a life of joy, connection, and resilience*? Join us on this extraordinary journey today. Email support@tweelie.com.au for more information

Resources

In Australia, various resources and organisations provide support and information for individuals with special needs and their families. Here are some essential resources:

National Disability Insurance Scheme (NDIS):
Website: NDIS
The NDIS provides support and services to Australians with disabilities, including financial assistance and access to various support providers.

Carers Australia:
Website: Carers Australia
Carers Australia offers support and resources for individuals caring for someone with a disability, including advocacy and information on available services.

Autism Spectrum Australia (Aspect):
Website: Autism Spectrum Australia
Aspect provides services, support, and resources for individuals on the autism spectrum and their families.

Cerebral Palsy Alliance:
Website: Cerebral Palsy Alliance
The Cerebral Palsy Alliance offers services and support for individuals with cerebral palsy and their families.

Down Syndrome Australia:
Website: Down Syndrome Australia
Down Syndrome Australia provides information, resources, and support for individuals with Down syndrome and their families.

Scope Australia:
Website: Scope Australia
Scope offers services and support for individuals with disabilities, including those with physical and intellectual disabilities.

Disability Discrimination Commissioner (Australian Human Rights Commission):
Website: Australian Human Rights Commission
The Disability Discrimination Commissioner promotes and protects the rights of people with disabilities, and the website provides information and resources.

Australian Coalition for Inclusive Education (ACIE):
Website: ACIE
ACIE advocates for inclusive education practices and provides resources for parents, educators, and policymakers. These organisations and resources cover a range of disabilities and provide valuable information, advocacy, and support for individuals with

special needs and their families in Australia. It is advisable to explore their websites or contact them directly for specific and up-to-date information.

Centrelink
Website: Centrelink

Centrelink is a government agency in Australia that provides services and financial assistance to eligible individuals and families. It operates under the Department of Human Services. Centrelink primarily focuses on delivering social security payments and services to Australians.

Medicare
Website: Medicare

Medicare is Australia's publicly funded universal health care system. It provides eligible Australian residents access to various medical services and hospital care at little to no cost. Medicare is administered by the Australian Government's Department of Human Services.

Notes

www.ingramcontent.com/pod-product-compliance
Lightning Source LLC
Chambersburg PA
CBHW030327080526
44584CB00012B/749